# Lyprinol

— • —

*A Natural Solution for*
*Arthritis and Other*
*Inflammatory Disorders*

## Georges Halpern, M.D., Ph.D.
Written with the collaboration of
Krista Edmonds, Ph.D.

AVERY
*a member of Penguin Putnam Inc. / New York*

Most Avery books are available at special quantity discounts for bulk purchases for sales promotions, premiums, fund-raising, and educational needs. Special books or book excerpts also can be created to fit specific needs. For details, write Putnam Special Markets, 375 Hudson Street, New York, NY 10014

AVERY

a member of
Penguin Putnam Inc.
375 Hudson Street
New York, NY 10014
*www.penguinputnam.com*

Library of Congress Cataloging-in-Publication Data

Halpern, Georges M.
Lyprinol : a natural solution for arthritis and other inflammatory disorders /
Georges Halpern ; written with the collaboration of Krista Edmonds.
p.   cm.
Includes bibliographical references and index.
ISBN 1-58333-103-4
1. Arthritis—alternative treatment.   2. Fish oils—therapeutic use.
3. Mussels.   4. Anti-inflammatory agents.   5. Omega-3 fatty acids—
Therapeutic use.   I. Edmonds, Krista.   II. Title. [DNLM: 1. Fatty Acids, Omega-3—therapeutic use.
2. Anti-inflammatory Agents, Non-steroidal—therapeutic use.   3. Arthritis—drug therapy.
4. Dietary Fats—therapeutic use.
QU 90 H195L 2000]
RC933 .H335     2000          2001022643
616.7'22061—dc21

Printed in the United States of America

1   3   5   7   9   10   8   6   4   2

# Acknowledgments

I must first thank all the physicians, scientists, nurses, and patients whose lives, experiences, and research made this book possible. Many thanks to my agent, Norman Goldfind, and Laura Shepherd, executive editor of Avery at Penguin Putnam, who had so much faith in me. Many thanks also to Robert L. Meyer and John D. Waitzer of Pharmalink International Ltd., who have supported my work with Lyprinol. Without Seemie Xavier, whose exceptional typing skills have made this writing process so much easier, this book would have been very difficult. And finally, so many, many thanks to my wife, Emiko, for her resilience, patience, and tolerance of the competing computer.

# Contents

# Lyprinol

# Introduction

*"Oh, my aching knees . . ."*

*"You know, it's just aging. The old joints begin to hurt."*

*"It's my arthritis, dear. I just can't knit or play the piano anymore."*

*"I don't remember the last time I went jogging. The arthritis is so bad."*

Do any of these statements sound familiar to you? If so, you're typical of millions of Americans who suffer from arthritis or who have helplessly watched the suffering of arthritic grandparents or parents. Perhaps you have tried over-the-counter or even prescription medication. But if you're like many others, you've found out that the benefits of these drugs are short-term at best. Worse, they are often fraught with unpleasant side effects.

"Isn't there a better way?" you've wondered.

This book is designed to show you a better way. It's a way that brings together the ancient legends and practices of a small New Zealand tribe and the discoveries and technological advances of today's most sophisticated scientists and manufacturers. This book will introduce you to Lyprinol, an oil derived from the green-lipped mussel.

# The Maori Legend

The Maoris are an ancient tribe native to New Zealand. They have claimed for centuries that consuming green-lipped mussels helps them maintain good health. The reported incidence of arthritis is extremely low among the coastal-dwelling Maoris, who consume large amounts of green-lipped mussels, whereas Maoris who reside in the interior areas of the country have the same incidence of arthritis as New Zealanders of European origin. This combination of ancient legend and careful observation of the Maoris' actual health patterns intrigued researchers in the United Kingdom, Australia, Austria, and Japan. They decided to investigate the mussels' reported anti-inflammatory activity. Eventually, the efforts of these researchers yielded Lyprinol—an oil extracted from green-lipped mussels once they have been freeze-dried into a stabilized powder.

Since the early 90s, clinical studies have shown that Lyprinol is highly effective as an anti-inflammatory agent in relieving symptoms of arthritis. These findings make sense, in light of earlier research into the biochemistry of inflammation. Researchers knew that marine lipids (the scientific word for fats) have long been used in medicine, and that they are actually the best and the most available source of fat in some areas of the world. They also knew that these marine lipids, regardless of their structure, have some protective effects on blood vessels and joints. They may even provide benefit to other organs such as the skin, the bronchi, and the gastrointestinal tract. The traditions of numerous varied populations confirm this scientific knowledge, maintaining that people who eat fatty fish enjoy better health. The benefits of fish oil were known not only in primitive but even in Western cultures. Your great-grandparents, for example, may have swallowed a spoonful of cod-liver oil before school or before bed. As a child, hiding in Savoie, France, during World War II, I also had cod-liver oil regularly—and loved it! We were not always sure of why it was beneficial; we just knew it was "good for us," and that it also tasted wonderful.

The benefits of fish oils aren't derived only from eating or drinking them. Topical application of fatty fish-oil concentrates can be beneficial to the skin, and have historically been used to remedy certain health problems—a fact that modern researchers are confirming. Cod-liver oil, for example, can help speed the healing of wounds. It may also prevent the formation of abnormal scars.

So why use Lyprinol, if cod-liver oil or other marine lipids will do? What's so special about the green-lipped mussel?

As the saying goes, we are what we eat. This statement is true for all living organisms, not merely for human beings. Even the tiny creatures that produce marine lipids are influenced by what *they* eat. Their diet consists of one-celled organisms called plankton. What's unusual about this particular population of plankton is that they are exposed to higher than normal levels of radiation, and that they have adapted by producing high levels of antioxidants to protect themselves. When the green-lipped mussels feed on this plankton, they absorb the same protection. So while all fish oils are beneficial, Lyprinol is higher in antioxidants than most others. Additionally, it is drawn from pure, pollution-free waters. The New Zealand government zealously protects the waters in which green-lipped mussels live, keeping them free of contaminants that affect fish from other regions of the world.

You don't necessarily have to use the oil extract to reap the health benefits of Lyprinol. You can eat the delicious green-lipped mussels as part of your daily diet. They are considered to be delicacies, and are sold all over the world. In fact, they are a staple in the best restaurants and fish markets around the globe. You don't need to worry about spoilage—the mussels are shipped live. If they are packed properly, they live up to three weeks without any problem.

Traditionally the Maori people have eaten them raw. You certainly can cook them if you prefer to do so, although they lose some of their nutritional benefits in the process. If you do not enjoy eating seafood products, have difficulty obtaining green-lipped mussels locally, or want more exact guidelines regarding quantities and dosages, you can buy Lyprinol in an already-existing preparation that yields as many health benefits as the raw or cooked mussel.

# The Varied Benefits of Lyprinol

Researchers have found that Lyprinol, which contains omega-3 polyunsaturated fatty acids (PUFAs), is one of the best anti-inflammatory agents available. Most chronic diseases that afflict people in Western society have an inflammatory component. Treatment options are not always ideal, and Lyprinol may be beneficial to many people who suffer from these diseases.

Arthritis, for example, costs Americans some $65 billion per year—almost 2.5 percent of the gross domestic product. Current research shows that both osteoarthritis and rheumatoid arthritis respond to Lyprinol with significant reductions in inflammation. Over 70 percent of patients studied reported relief, and up to 98 percent reported a reduction in swelling. Moreover, Lyprinol has been found to be nontoxic and free of significant side effects. Unlike most medications used to treat arthritis—such as nonsteroidal anti-inflammatory drugs (NSAIDs), which have adverse gastrointestinal side effects—the lipid extract of green-lipped mussel actually *protects* the gastrointestinal tract.

Other than its positive anti-inflammatory effects, Lyprinol is also helpful in the prevention and treatment of cardiovascular problems. This is true of other fish oils as well. However, Lyprinol is considered to be safer than other fish oils for those with circulatory problems. Other fish oils can sometimes cause excessive bleeding in case of injury because they inhibit blood clotting, but Lyprinol doesn't affect the platelets in the blood that are responsible for clotting. This means that it's completely safe for menstruating women, or for patients who are already taking blood thinners such as aspirin.

Lyprinol shows promise as an antiasthma and antiallergy treatment. Asthma affects an estimated seventeen million Americans—more than 6 percent of the population—including nearly five million children. The disease is responsible for nearly half a million hospitalizations, more than one million emergency room visits, and more than five thousand deaths annually, at a cost of approximately $6.2 billion per year. Sobering statistics indeed.

Studies around the world have shown that Lyprinol reduces asthma symptoms, due to its anti-inflammatory effects on airways leading to the lungs. It also has been found to be safer than today's frequently used pharmaceuticals—including the new antileukotriene medications that are supposed to be relatively free of side effects.

Even the skin can benefit from Lyprinol, which protects against radiation and also slows the skin's natural aging process. The carotenoids and omega-3 fatty acids present in Lyprinol are essential for healthy skin. Like other fish oils, which contain essential fatty acids associated with skin protection, Lyprinol speeds wound healing and prevents excessive scarring.

Here are some fascinating possibilities associated with Lyprinol. Most are still under investigation, but are worth discussing because they have such enormous potential. For example, Lyprinol may actually strengthen your response to the influenza vaccine! Some studies suggest that Lyprinol may prevent cancer in laboratory animals, and formal studies using human subjects are currently under way. And inflammatory digestive disorders such as Crohn's disease and ulcerative colitis may well respond to the anti-inflammatory properties of Lyprinol. The potential effectiveness of Lyprinol in the therapy of inflammatory bowel diseases opens a variety of exciting doors to future treatments.

Further research will help to expand our understanding of Lyprinol's health benefits. This book will discuss what we know now and how that knowledge can enhance your health.

# How This Book Can Help You

If you are suffering from any inflammatory disorder, Lyprinol can help you. After giving you a brief glimpse into the history and characteristics of Lyprinol, we will review the recent research on green-lipped mussel extracts as well as technical issues surrounding the development of stable mussel preparations.

Chapters 3 and 4 will look at inflammatory diseases in general and arthritis in particular, and will show how Lyprinol can be effective in reducing symptoms of rheumatoid as well as osteoarthritis. Chapter 5 will focus on the effects of Lyprinol on the cardiovascular system, and chapter 6 will discuss its effectiveness in addressing asthma, allergies, and skin disorders. Chapter 7 looks at the needs of women, specifically addressing how Lyprinol can be helpful in alleviating menstrual discomforts. Chapter 8 offers a tantalizing glimpse into the future by reviewing research currently under way into new applications of this extraordinary oil. Chapter 9 will provide guidelines in how to use Lyprinol.

# 1

•

# The History
# of Lyprinol

Let's begin by taking a brief look at Lyprinol—what it is, where it comes from, and how it was introduced to the Western world.

## Meet *Perna Canaliculus*

No, this is not a Latin lesson. You're being formally introduced to the green-lipped mussel, using its correct biological name, *Perna canaliculus,* which—like all scientific names of living creatures—is Latin. Lyprinol is the new patented, stabilized natural marine lipid extract from the New Zealand green-lipped mussel. It contains a rare combination of lipid groups containing both known and unknown polyunsaturated fatty acids (PUFAs). You'll learn more about these

PUFAs later on. For now, let's just say that the known PUFAs, which include omega-3s and some eicosatetraenoic acids (ETAs), have been shown to be extremely powerful anti-inflammatory compounds that are particularly effective against arthritis.

Why is Lyprinol so effective? Given the plenitude of local fish and their oils, many of which help in reducing inflammation, why search for a product imported from the exotic waters of New Zealand?

The answer is that Lyprinol is a purer product than most fish oils because the green-lipped mussel lives in such a sheltered and protected environment. But it isn't just the pollution-free waters that make Lyprinol a superior marine oil. The lipids found in Lyprinol are especially rich and efficacious. These developed through a combination of the mussels' genetics and their food—tiny organisms called microplankton. The planktons are rich in antioxidants because of the amount of sunlight that falls upon the waters where they live. The sun's rays are unusually intense and in order to survive, these planktons must protect themselves from the high levels of ultraviolet (UV) radiation, which can reach potentially deadly levels. The planktons on which the mussels feed have evolved to fight oxidative stress caused by radiation. The mussels, in turn, absorb the protective mechanisms. When you eat the mussels—or their extracted oil—you ingest the wonderful protective properties of the planktons. Now they can protect *you* against all sorts of conditions you'll learn more about later in this book.

# How Did This Well-Kept Secret Arrive in the West?

The answer to this lies in a history lesson that goes back many centuries. About one thousand years ago, the Maoris arrived in New Zealand. It appears that they began to consume large quantities of green-lipped mussels during the fifteenth century, when an extended cold period forced them to spend whole summers fishing along the coast and smoke-drying their catches for storage. When the climate warmed up again (approximately during the sixteenth century), heavy rainfall and gale-force winds increased flooding and made life on the coast uncomfortable. It appears that as they moved farther inland, they retained their taste for seafood.

Their strong attachment to the green-lipped mussel, however, was not merely a matter of taste. They believed, as modern-day Maoris continue to believe, that consuming these mussels helped them maintain good health. Today, we know that their belief was no mere superstition, and that there are scientifically proven reasons for their good health.

Europeans started to arrive in New Zealand in the mid-1600s, beginning with Abel Tasman and Captain Cook. After this, the flow of Europeans never stopped. When European settlers began to arrive in New Zealand in significant numbers during the nineteenth century, they brought with them their European diseases as well as their bad health habits, including the European diet, and the use of alcohol and tobacco.

The Maori population fell from about 120,000 in 1769 to 42,000 in 1896. A major factor in their dwindling numbers was poor resistance to diseases such as smallpox, influenza, German measles, tuberculosis, whooping cough, typhoid, and sexually transmitted diseases. Medical assistance was scarce. Even when sparse medical resources could be marshalled, they usually reached the rural Maoris too late to save lives.

Maoris also succumbed to alcohol abuse and experienced all its resultant problems. The introduction of the musket added a new devastation to the Maoris' own land battles. By the late nineteenth century, the European settlers were referring to the Maoris as "a dying race."

While most Maoris soon fell prey to European ailments, coastal Maoris appeared to be healthier. In particular, they did not suffer from arthritis as their European counterparts did. Anecdotal evidence and folk wisdom attribute this health benefit to the heavy consumption of raw green-lipped mussels.

# The Maori Secret and Western Science

Interest in the green-lipped mussel began when it was noticed that the coastal Maoris had far less arthritis than the inland Maoris. A company from Australia began investigating the health benefits of the New Zealand green-lipped mussel in the 1970s and spearheaded the pioneering work that eventually led to the production of Lyprinol. Their goal was to prove the effectiveness of a green-lipped mussel product, and then manufacture and deliver that product and its natural health benefits to arthritis sufferers and other health-conscious consumers. They have succeeded in accomplishing that goal.

The first products produced from the New Zealand green-lipped mussel were various preparations of dried mussel powder. These preparations were less than ideal. They were unstable; they held residual moisture, and they had a characteristic odor that many people found offensive.

By 1975, a new freeze-dried powder extract became available. It was less malodorous and therefore became considerably more popular. However, hard scientific evidence supporting the product's popularity was still lacking. By 1978, manufacturers of the mussel extract were actively seeking scientific validation of their claims that their extract could be helpful in reducing symptoms of arthritis. They succeeded in piquing the interest of Drs. Robin Gibson and Sheila Gibson, a Scottish husband-and-wife medical team, who conducted the first major study. Their results, published in the *Practitioner* in 1980, showed clearly that the mussel extract had a substantial effect on certain forms of arthritis.

Unfortunately the Gibsons' results, though promising, were not easily replicated. The discrepancy between study findings turned out to be caused by the fact that the clinical studies utilized unstable mussel powder. Today, the stabilized powder is readily available and is the superior product.

It is important to note that many scientific studies that have not found mussel powder to be effective have used the unstable, rather than the stabilized, powder. This is an understandable error, since the European manufacturers, who sell unstabilized powder, use the same brand name—Seatone®—as the Australian and Japanese manufacturers who use stabilized powder. The unstable product has given Lyprinol a bad reputation. Until 1983, researchers studying the effects of the mussel extract experienced considerable variations in the level of anti-inflammatory activity from batch to batch due to poor stability.

The last chapter of this book will tell you where and how you can obtain the highest quality Lyprinol.

# Further Research

The Australian company, convinced that the mussels contained some potent active ingredient, began research to identify what that ingredient might be and to isolate it. In 1992, Dr. W. Henry Betts, the principal scientist at the Rheumatology Research Laboratory of the Queen Elizabeth Hospital in South Australia, discovered some very active compounds in mussel extract. Dr. Betts had previously established an *in vitro* method of testing anti-inflammatory compounds. He was amazed to discover that some of the compounds extracted from the green-lipped mussel were the most potent in his laboratory! Unfortunately, they were not pure enough for him to identify them.

His interest had been captured, however, and he was not willing to let the implications of these findings slip away from him. His enthusiasm led him to introduce the Australian entrepreneurs of the New Zealand mussel to Dr. Michael W. Whitehouse, an expert in testing for anti-inflammatory activity in laboratory animals. In 1994 Dr. Whitehouse's laboratory animal studies confirmed the activity that Dr. Betts had shown in his testing.

# How Lyprinol Is Produced

Welcome to Germany, where mussels are transformed into a product that can help you wake up in the morning without creaking or pain in your joints.

How does this happen? Let's go back to Dr. Betts and Dr. Whitehouse.

Having identified the area in which activity existed, the next question was how the lipids identified by Dr. Betts could be extracted commercially without damaging the active compounds. It took two more years of intensive testing to develop the protocols for the patented process, which utilizes liquefied carbon dioxide instead of chemical solvents to extract the pure lipids. They are then combined with pharmaceutical-grade olive oil, encapsulated . . . and *voilà!* We have Lyprinol.

The production of Lyprinol has become a smooth, technologically advanced, and seamless process. The mussels are harvested from the pristine waters of the Marlborough Sound of New Zealand by specifically equipped ships that are totally enclosed so they release no pollution. In less than two hours, the mussels—which are kept under maximum refrigeration to ensure freshness—reach the grinder and centrifuge at the factory. They go through a series of processes to extract their essential liquid, which is combined with stabilizing tartaric acid and freeze-dried. The result: Seatone, a freeze-dried, stabilized powder of mussel. It is produced using Good Manufacturing Practices, as defined by the pharmaceutical industry and approved by the United States Food and Drug Administration. Seatone is then shipped to Germany, where the oil is extracted by a supercritical liquid carbon dioxide process. The end product is Lyprinol, a patent-protected, suitably concentrated, and stabilized dietary supplement.

Once processed from Seatone, Lyprinol does not contain any salt and can be safely used by patients with high blood pressure, or anyone adhering to a low-sodium diet. Lyprinol contains no carbohydrates, making it safe for diabetics; nor does it contain any protein. Finally, Lyprinol is easily digestible.

Now that you know something about the characteristics and history of Lyprinol, let's have a look at how it actually works.

# 2

•

# The Science
# of Lyprinol

Can diet influence disease? The idea of a connection between what we eat and how healthy we are has been explored throughout history in numerous cultures, both primitive and modern. Obviously, ancient peoples understood that eating certain foods—say, poisonous mushrooms—led to acute illnesses or death. But even among the ancients, myths and legends abounded regarding the impact of diet on health. In today's world, the connection between diet and chronic illnesses such as heart disease and diabetes is obvious and wholly accepted in popular and scientific circles. *Cholesterol* and *low blood sugar,* for example, have become household words.

Only in the last two or three decades, however, have scientists become aware of the connection between diet and other diseases. Researchers are linking diet to cancer as well as to inflammatory diseases. They are discovering that lifestyle and diet are even more important than family history. Studies of immigrants show that the rate of disease among populations changes as their environment changes. Their new lifestyles are probably as important as their genetic profile.

A good example of this is the incidence of heart disease and breast cancer among the Japanese. Japanese people living in their own country and adhering to their traditional diet—which is low in animal fats and high in brown rice and proteins such as tofu—have relatively few cases of heart disease and breast cancer. Japanese people living in Hawaii who have included more "American" foods in their diet have a higher incidence of these diseases, while Japanese living on the West Coast of the United States have the highest incidence of all. This disturbing trend is clearly related to the Americanization of their diet.

While America is purported to be the wealthiest country in the world, that affluence has not translated itself into better health. Quite the contrary. Our sedentary lifestyle, combined with the easy availability of foods high in animal fat, sugars, and chemicals, has led to an array of diseases. Cardiovascular disease, cancer, and arthritis top the list. However, other conditions are rising significantly. These include rheumatoid arthritis, multiple sclerosis, chronic fatigue syndrome, inflammatory bowel disorders (such as ulcerative colitis and Crohn's disease), some forms of diabetes, fibromyalgia, lupus erythematosus, some thyroid disorders, and scleroderma. These are called autoimmune disorders. They arise when your immune system starts attacking structures within your own body.

Western science has fought back with an impressive array of immunosuppressive drugs designed to suppress the immune system. While they are effective in controlling serious flare-ups of symptoms, they also cause almost as many problems as they solve. Suppressing your immune system means that you're more vulnerable to invasions of viruses and bacteria. The drugs can also damage healthy organs. And ultimately, they don't solve the problem. They merely relieve the symptoms for a little while—and only as long as you take them.

Solid scientific research has begun to point us in the direction of lifestyle changes that *can* solve the problem—or at least contribute to its solution. Reducing consumption of animal fats and increasing dietary intake of vegetables, fruits, and whole grains decrease the inflammation that occurs in many autoimmune disorders. Eating deep-water fish instead of hamburgers, hydrogenated oils, and high-fat cheeses may make your joints less achy.

All oils are not created equal, and all fat isn't bad. You may be surprised to learn that some fats are necessary for good health. Scientists have found that supplementing the diet with oils high in certain essential fatty acids (such as omega-3 and some omega-6) is highly beneficial. Some of these "good" oils are plant based. These include flaxseed, rapeseed, borage, evening primrose, and canola oils. Small amounts of these "good" oils are also present in baked beans and most green leafy vegetables. Other healthful oils are fish based. Cod-liver oil is perhaps the best-known example, but there are others as well.

Even among these beneficial oils, some are superior to others. When scientists compared the effects of dietary supplementation with fish oil to dietary supplementation with flaxseed oil, they found that marine and vegetable oils were very similar in some of their beneficial effects. However, they also discovered that the omega-3 PUFAs contained in fish were five to ten times more efficacious than the omega-3 PUFAs found in plants! This means that very large amounts of flaxseed oil were needed to accomplish what relatively small quantities of marine oil managed to do—namely, to reduce elevated *triacylglycerol* levels in the blood. Triacylglycerols are lipids found in the blood. Excessively high levels place a person at risk for diabetes and cardiovascular disease.

Let's look more closely at some of the scientific research supporting the benefits of fish oils in general and Lyprinol in particular.

# The Scientific Study of Marine Lipids

The growing body of evidence about the beneficial effects of omega-3 fatty acids makes it increasingly clear that fish is a much more important food than had previously been supposed. But scientists didn't come to this conclusion by jumping directly to a study of fish. They began by looking at PUFAs in general. American researchers identified two major categories of PUFAs as far back as the 1930s. They were called omega-6 and omega-3 acids. It was discovered that *linoleic acid* is the parent or precursor for the omega-6 PUFAs, while *alpha-linolenic acid* is the parent fatty acid for the omega-3 PUFAs. Research continued into the various health benefits—and possible drawbacks—of each category.

Let's jump an ocean and several decades and drop in on two Danish scientists named H.O. Bang and J. Dyerberg. In 1972, they noticed that the Inuits of Greenland had a much lower incidence of death from coronary heart disease and other diseases associated with affluence than other citizens of Greenland, despite a diet consisting mainly of seal fat. In addition, their blood fat levels were relatively low—a surprising finding, considering their high-fat diet. In fact, their entire blood profile reflected a picture of good health, especially compared with Danes from Greenland whose diet was "Western." Bang and Dyerberg were baffled. These findings flew in the face of established beliefs about cholesterol levels and their effects on coronary heart disease. How could anyone live on seal fat and have such idyllic cholesterol and triglyceride levels? And why weren't the Inuits suffering from heart attacks?

After much research, the two scientists concluded that the low incidence of heart disease could be attributed to the Inuits' marine diet. They showed that the unusual blood lipid profile of Greenland Inuits was consistent with reductions in heart attacks. They began to draw connections to other cultures and countries. For example, they noted that incidence of heart disease and resulting death fell dramatically in Norway following the German invasion in 1940, when the Norwegians shifted to a fish-based rather than a meat-based diet. Since the pioneering work of Bang and Dyerberg, scientists have studied dozens of other cultures throughout the world. Again and again, findings confirm the association between a high-fish diet and a low incidence of cardiovascular disease.

# A Closer Look at Fat

Remember our discussion of omega-6 and omega-3 PUFAs? Let's take a closer look at these, so as to understand why the fats that dominate our Western diet tend to be so destructive, while fish-based fats are so healing. It is especially important to understand more about the science of fats because the subject has become a source of great confusion during recent decades.

As we enter the twenty-first century, the type of dietary fat required for optimum health has become a confusing subject not only for consumers but even for scientists. In fact, it is a controversial subject all around. I have heard people say that every few months, they turn on their televisions and encounter reports of some scientific finding concerning fat that appears to contradict the last finding.

There is a historical basis for all the confusion. Although fats and oils have been part of the human diet since the beginning of recorded time, scientific study of dietary lipids lagged behind the study of proteins and carbohydrates during the development of nutritional science in the eighteenth century. In fact, fat was not even recognized as an important nutrient until 1827. Only in the 1900s was fat recognized as a source of abundant energy, as well as a vehicle for the metabolism of four major fat-soluble vitamins. The concept of "essential fatty acids" is a relatively recent phenomenon.

As Western consumption of animal fat (mainly lard and butter) increased dramatically through the beginning of the twentieth century, the study of fat became more urgent and rose to prominence in the scientific world. Epidemiologists began correlating high levels of serum cholesterol with prevalence of coronary heart disease. Because of their urging, people began altering their diet. They reduced consumption of animal fats and switched to other fats that supposedly were less destructive. Margarine was touted as a healthful alternative to butter, for example. People began to believe that if they avoided egg yolks and red meat, nibbling instead on margarine sandwiches, they would have a healthy blood profile. The main PUFA in the Western food supply became linoleic acid, the precursor of the omega-6 series, and the major fatty acid found in most vegetable oils. The "solution" generated unforeseen consequences, however, leading to an entirely new set of problems.

The main problem was that people were now consuming large quantities of omega-6 fatty acids. This fatty acid is not in and of itself destructive. In fact, it is very effective at lowering blood cholesterol levels. What is destructive, however, is that we eat so much of it—and so little of the other primary class of PUFAs, known as the omega-3 series. These are equally essential, but are not present at very high levels in most Western diets.

Large quantities of omega-6 fatty acids created a new imbalance in our dietary fats. The high level of omega-6 relative to omega-3 PUFAs in the Western diet (a ratio of about 15:1 or higher!) is due to

a diet enriched in linoleic acid from sources such as marga
salad oils. Prior to the widespread use of omega 6–rich vege
in the food supply, the omega-6/omega-3 ratio in diets was closer to
1:1. Consumption of these oils has risen dramatically—and, ironi-
cally, because people believe that these fats are good for their health.
This, however, isn't true and the glut of omega-6 vegetable oils has
caused a sharp rise in cardiovascular disease.

The key concept is *balance*. Let's look at this concept more
closely.

# A Balancing Act

The balance between the omega-6 and omega-3 essential fatty acids
has become increasingly central to our understanding of good
health. Both groups serve as precursors for a host of chemicals that
perform necessary functions in our body. A precursor is a chemical
that precedes or "parents" another chemical. Chemical #2 is derived
from chemical #1. Some of the chemicals that are derived from the
omega-6 and omega-3 groups are prostaglandins, prostacyclins,
thromboxanes, and leukotrienes. All these complicated-sounding
substances are crucial to our good health. They affect our immune
systems, our circulatory systems, and our joints. When they are cor-
rectly balanced, we remain healthy. Our joints do not become inflamed. The membranes in our airways also remain free of
inflammation so we do not suffer from asthma. The mucosal lining
in our digestive tract is protected, so we do not suffer from irritable
bowel syndrome, or other inflammatory digestive disorders. Our
blood fat (cholesterol and triglyceride) levels are healthy, and we do

not suffer from as many heart attacks, strokes, or other cardiovascular problems. Our circulation remains normal, and we don't suffer from thrombosis.

How does this balance work?

Let's look at each type of PUFA. The omega-6 group contains large quantities of *linoleic acid* (LA). This is the precursor chemical for *arachidonic acid* which, in turn, leads to the production of many other chemicals. When these chemicals are overproduced, they can have negative effects. The omega-3 group, on the other hand, is rich in *alpha-linolenic acid* (ALA), which is a precursor to two other EFAs— *eicosapentaenoic acid* (EPA) and *docosahexaenoic acid* (DHA). These have the opposite effect of arachidonic acid. They inhibit production of the substances that arachidonic acid generally stimulates.

The system of checks and balances works quite well. Arachidonic acid causes the production of important substances, while EPA and DHA make sure that these substances are not overproduced.

Let's look at a few examples of this balance in action.

Scientists studying thrombosis—a condition that occurs when a blood clot is lodged within a blood vessel—discovered that the key to maintaining healthy blood vessels lies in maintaining a balance between two chemicals in the body. One, called thromboxane 2 ($TXA_2$), causes blood cells to clump together and blood vessels to tighten and constrict. We need this substance so that when we cut ourselves, our blood will clot and a scab will form. Constricted blood vessels reduce the amount of blood that reaches the area, thereby minimizing blood loss.

On the other hand, we don't want blood clots moving through our arteries and veins. They are very dangerous. They block the flow of blood, causing numerous problems at the site of the clot. Even worse, they travel. A blood clot that reaches the heart can be fatal. So the body balances out the $TXA_2$ by producing another chemical called prostacyclin ($PGI_2$). This works against the clotting of blood and also promotes dilation, or widening, of the blood vessels.

For us to remain healthy, a correct balance of both these chemicals must be maintained. Thrombosis occurs when the balance is disrupted. $TXA_2$ is not counterbalanced by sufficient quantities of $PGI_2$. One of the exciting discoveries about the Greenland Inuits was that their blood is rich in EPA, which plays an important role in maintaining the balance between $TXA_2$ and $PGI_2$. The Danes, on the other hand, hardly had any detectable levels of EPA in their blood at all!

Researchers have since established that increased consumption of fish oil leads to increased production of $PGI_2$, resulting in the remarkable lack of thrombosis and other circulatory difficulties among the Eskimos. We will encounter more examples of the role that the omega-3 oils play in balancing out the effects of the omega-6 category as we delve further into the benefits of Lyprinol.

As mentioned above, marine-based omega-3 oils have been shown to be superior to plant-based oils. Their benefits are associated not only with preventing cardiovascular disease but also with reduction in inflammatory disorders, such as arthritis. For example, arachidonic acid leads to the production of leukotrienes. These are beneficial substances, and they accomplish a host of necessary functions in the body. Believe it or not, inflammation is an example of a necessary function. It is your body's way of fighting unwelcome and potentially dangerous invading organisms. Too many leukotrienes, however, lead to unnecessary and counterproductive inflammation. Inflammatory disorders such as arthritis, asthma, and irritable bowel syndrome are all associated with excessive production of leukotrienes.

Omega-3 PUFAs control leukotriene production, leading to a reduction in inflammation. As we'll see below, all the omega-3 PUFAs are helpful in inhibiting leukotrienes, but fish oil is more efficacious than plant-based oil. Lyprinol is the most powerful anti-inflammatory marine oil available at present.

# All Fish Oils Are Not Created Equal

As we have seen, fish oil is highly beneficial. But all fish oils are not equally beneficial. Let's look at the most recent research on the subject.

The marine food chain is dominated by omega-3 PUFAs. Fish, shellfish, and other fish products such as fish eggs (roe) or oils such as cod-liver oil are the main sources of fish-based omega-3 PUFAs in our diet. Research has shown that Lyprinol is superior to oils derived from fish and roe—and even to oils derived from other shellfish.

The secret lies in Lyprinol's unique ingredients. It has properties not found in any other marine lipid sources. In fact, it is two hundred times more effective at reducing swelling of arthritic paws in laboratory animals than other fish oils that contain more run-of-the-mill PUFAs. The active ingredients of Lyprinol are a series of unique omega-3 PUFAs called ETAs. A critical review conducted at two separate universities in Australia found that these ingredients are responsible for Lyprinol's uniqueness. Lyprinol stands alone in its ability to successfully suppress leukotrienes, which are responsible for initiating and spreading inflammation throughout the body.

We have all heard of inflammation, but what exactly is it? Inflammation is one of the ways in which the body controls infection and promotes healing. In the right context, the body's ability to produce inflammation is actually critical to good health. But you can also have too much of a good thing—at which point it stops being a good thing and becomes a problem. In the case of arthritis, asthma, and similar conditions, the process goes awry and the body fights itself. It sends out its inflammatory "soldiers" to fight interior "friends" instead of invading external "enemies." Conditions such as rheumatoid arthritis and asthma are therefore called autoimmune diseases— the body is producing "immunity" against itself.

Leukotrienes, chemicals that cause inflammation, are released by healthy individuals to combat illness. But those who suffer from autoimmune diseases produce too many leukotrienes. These chemicals develop through the *LOX pathway.* No, that's not the road to a delicious Sunday morning bagel. LOX stands for *lipoxygenase,* and it is one of two major pathways responsible for inflammation. The other is called *COX,* which stands for *cyclo-oxygenase.* Both these pathways function through producing a chemical called *arachidonate,* which is responsible for oxygenization (the addition of oxygen to form a new substance). The new substances formed by the LOX pathway are the leukotrienes. The COX pathway produces other inflammatory substances, called prostaglandins and thromboxanes. When either or both of these pathways malfunction, producing excessive leukotrienes, prostaglandins, or thromboxanes, inflammation results. You wake up groaning with arthritic pain, or wheezing with asthma, for example.

Current anti-inflammatory medications, the NSAIDs (see Appendix B for a current list), function by inhibiting the COX pathway. As mentioned, these drugs can have serious side effects. What's more, they don't address inflammatory activity caused by the LOX pathway. So scientists are turning their attention to developing inhibitors of the LOX pathway. A new class of drugs called antileukotrienes is being used to address asthma, for example. However, these do not address COX activity. Many asthmatics need to take several different medications, with an array of side effects. Is there a substance that can inhibit *both* the LOX and the COX pathways? The answer is yes. Lyprinol appears to inhibit both these inflammatory pathways—quite a feat for a single substance.

Lyprinol's wide range of impressive results can be attributed to the fact that it actually is *not* a single substance. Indeed, there are a variety of active ingredients contained in Lyprinol, over and above the fatty acids that have so far been identified. For example, there are about ten different marine sterols (a kind of oil) and more than thirty different fatty acids in Lyprinol. These are mixtures of all kinds of fats—saturated, monounsaturated, and polyunsaturated. Each of these ingredients has a different effect on an aspect of the COX or LOX pathway.

For example, three particular unsaturated fatty acids present in Lyprinol have emerged as new, previously unidentified substances that work against arachidonate. These are called *antimetabolites*, because they work against the metabolism of arachidonate. They work synergistically together with other oils, such as EPA and DHA, which are present in many marine foods as well as Lyprinol. The result is an amazingly powerful combination of chemicals that inhibit metabolism of arachidonates produced by *both* pathways. Perhaps this is the reason why smaller quantities of Lyprinol are required to bring about anti-inflammatory results. There are more fatty acids present, and they all strengthen and enhance one another's effectiveness.

The unusual fatty acids present in Lyprinol also appear to be best suited to suppressing the production of leukotrienes because of their unusual structure. One particular omega-3 fatty acid, called omega-3 tetraenoic, is virtually identical to arachidonic acid, which is the agent responsible for acting on the COX and LOX pathways to produce inflammation. This acid can "fool" the pathways into "believing" that they are bonding with arachidonic acid, with the happy result that inflammatory agents, such as leukotrienes, are not produced.

# No Side Effects

You might think that such a potent and far-reaching substance would have distressing side effects. The bonus is that Lyprinol is free of these effects. It appears that the fatty acids in Lyprinol can distinguish between different aspects of the COX pathway and target only those responsible for inflammation. The COX pathway actually consists of two components—COX-1 and COX-2. COX-1 is a "housekeeper." It is responsible for upkeep of the areas in the body that have protective mucous linings—including the digestive tract. COX-2 is responsible for inflammation. Unlike NSAIDs, Lyprinol suppresses COX-2, while leaving COX-1 untouched. So there are no unpleasant digestive side effects.

The stomach isn't the only region of the body that is safe from side effects. In fact, all areas of the body are safe when you take Lyprinol. You can't really overdose on it, either. Dr. Whitehouse of Australia tried his best to induce some kind of negative reaction in mice by giving them megadoses of Lyprinol. He didn't manage to kill even a single mouse.

So it works, and it's safe. But don't take my word for it. Let's look at some of the scientific studies supporting these statements.

# A Review of Scientific Studies

Many scientific studies have focused on Lyprinol. Most of these studies unequivocally support the effectiveness of Lyprinol, and many point to its superiority not only over conventional medications and plant-based omega-3 PUFAs, but even over other marine oils. Let's look at a few of these studies.

- A double-blind study conducted at Glasgow Hospital in Scotland found that Lyprinol inhibited leukotriene synthesis, reducing the severity of one particular form of arthritis in laboratory rats.

- Studies conducted at Queen Elisabeth Hospital in Adelaide, Australia, demonstrated that Lyprinol inhibits activity of the LOX pathway, reducing the damaging effects of persistent inflammation and bringing relief to those who suffer from various allergic reactions, including asthma. The studies also supported the effectiveness of Lyprinol in bringing about relief from arthritis symptoms.

- A study conducted at the University of Queensland in Australia tested the antiarthritis properties of Lyprinol by measuring a series of arthritis symptoms in laboratory rats. Lyprinol reduced joint swelling by 91 percent, compared to untreated rats, which experienced no reduction in swelling at all. Lyprinol was 200 to 350 times as effective as other oils used to treat inflammation—at one-hundredth the dosage!

As if these findings were not outstanding enough, the University of Queensland scientists compared Lyprinol with indomethacin and ibuprofen—two widely used anti-arthritic drugs. At the same dose rate, Lyprinol outperformed both by a factor of two to one.

- A randomized clinical trial of Lyprinol was conducted in Scotland. It involved sixty patients. Thirty participants suffered from classic rheumatoid arthritis. The other thirty had clinical and radiological evidence of osteoarthritis. Both groups of patients showed significant improvement with Lyprinol. Over 70 percent of all participants who completed the trial benefited from being included in the trial.

- A pilot study conducted in Denmark on patients suffering from osteoarthritis showed that Lyprinol dramatically decreased the level of pain in a two- to three-month period.

- Further studies compared Lyprinol to other oils claiming to have antiarthritic properties—flaxseed oil, evening primrose oil, salmon oil, and Max-EPA® (a fish-oil product). The researchers used an equal dosage of each oil and measured the effect of each agent in controlling joint swelling associated with arthritis. Lyprinol proved to be:

  - 200 times more potent than Max-EPA
  - 250 times more potent than unprocessed green-lipped mussel extract
  - 350 times more potent than evening primrose oil
  - 350 times more potent than salmon oil
  - 400 times more potent than flaxseed oil

The combined findings of all these studies point to Lyprinol as the most effective agent in reducing arthritis symptoms. It is superior to conventional pharmaceuticals, vegetable-based omega-3 oils, other fish oils, and even unprocessed extract of the green-lipped mussel.

# Balancing Your Own Fat Intake

There are two different approaches to oils. One focuses on the amount of oils consumed, and the other looks at the types of oils consumed. Certainly it is valuable to examine how much oil you're actually consuming on a regular basis. Do you cook with oil? Do you incorporate it into cakes and breads? Do you use spreads, such as butter or margarine, which are fatty? Is fat a favorite ingredient of your salad dressing? You can tally up how much oil you ingest by estimating how many tablespoons you eat every day from all these varied sources. Many studies have shown that a high-fat diet contributes to cancer, cardiovascular disease, and a host of other dangerous conditions.

But don't go to the other extreme and completely shun all fat. Remember that you need essential fatty acids, which are not produced by your own body. You need both omega-6 and omega-3 fatty acids. But you don't need to pour enormous quantities of oil into your mouth—or your frying pan. Remember that fatty acids work like medicine in your system. When you take a drug, you don't take huge quantities. You usually can swallow a small pill, containing just the right quantity of active ingredients. These powerful substances shoot through your body like missiles. They go right to your body's receptors and do their job, creating appropriate reactions in your body.

You know that you can take excessive quantities of some substances, such as certain vitamins, and suffer no ill effects. If you take too much vitamin C, for example, the excess is simply excreted in your urine. However, you know that many medications can have serious and even life-threatening consequences when taken in excess. Fats should be regarded as "medications" that can be unhealthful when taken in excess. Sure, the part you need is absorbed and used by the body, but the excess is not excreted. Rather, it is stored. Some is stored in your body's cells. This is the part that contributes to unsightly weight problems. Some is stored along and within blood vessels, contributing to atherosclerosis. You don't want to eat too much fat, nor do you want to completely eliminate fat. The key is to eat healthful fats in appropriate quantities and in correct balance.

Let's look at the physiology of most natural fats. If you shine a light through a slide of fat in liquid form or in a very thin solid form, the light will be diverted. If the light moves toward you, it's called a *cis*-fatty acid. However, if you hydrogenate or heat your oils, the light moves away from you and you get a *trans*-fatty acid.

The trans-fatty acids have been shown to be irritants. In fact, they are pro-inflammatory—*if* they are consumed by themselves. Margarine or most shortenings are trans-fatty acids. Baked goods contain lots of trans-fatty acids because they become solid at room temperature and resist heat very well. When they are absorbed and metabolized, they give rise to more arachidonic acid precursors. Remember that these are, in turn, the precursors of inflammatory substances. Self-standing trans-fatty acids also create damage to the inner layer of your small arteries. This is the initial stage for creating inflammation of the artery that will eventually lead to cardiovascular disease.

It's hard to get away from these fats. They seem to be present in just about everything—especially our favorite foods. However, it is crucial to cut down on them because of their destructive effects. This does not mean that we have to completely eliminate them. If we reduce our trans-fatty acids and substitute cis-fatty acids, we are tipping the balance toward the healthier side. Try to use unprocessed, expeller-pressed oils—especially *monounsaturated* oils, such as olive and canola. These work nicely alone, and even better in combination. Canola oil can be heated at a much higher temperature than olive oil without becoming bitter and potentially toxic.

Just as important, using these oils will help counterbalance your intake of omega-6 fatty acids by increasing your intake of omega-3 fatty acids. These will offset some of the negative results of the trans-fatty acids. They will also provide the balance we discussed earlier between the categories of omega-6 and omega-3 acids so that they function most optimally in your body.

Some research has suggested that there is metabolic competition between omega-3 and omega-6 PUFAs, as if each is trying to "elbow" the other aside and claim its place in the sun. The implication is that omega-6 PUFAs derived from vegetable oils could actually reduce the efficacy of omega-3 PUFAs in fish oil and hence weaken the power of fish oil to reduce cardiovascular disease. These findings appeared to suggest that presence of excessive vegetable-based omega-6 oils weakens the power of the omega-3 PUFAs derived from fish. Later findings, however, implied that any quantity of fish oil will have some beneficial impact on levels of fats present in the blood, and therefore offer some degree of protection against cardiovascular disease. But remember optimum benefits will be derived from eating a proper balance between omega-3 and omega-6 PUFAs.

Now you have been introduced to different types of fatty acids. You know the difference between trans- and cis-fatty acids, and between the omega-6 and the omega-3 groups. You are also familiar with research pointing to the superiority of fish oil in general, and

Lyprinol in particular. Let's have a closer look at a typical Lyprinol capsule. What's in it? And how should you use it?

# What's in a Lyprinol Capsule?

An exhaustive catalogue with detailed explanations of all the ingredients in each Lyprinol capsule is beyond the purview of this book. In this section, we will review the main ingredients. Details are provided in Appendix A.

*Mussel oil:* Each Lyprinol capsule consists of 50 milligrams of mussel oil. Because pure mussel oil is very sticky and very difficult to handle, it is mixed with 100 milligrams of pharmaceutical-grade olive oil, yielding two parts of olive oil and one part of Lyprinol. This may sound like a large quantity of oil but, actually, it's not. In one experiment, patients were given up to fifty capsules of Lyprinol a day—which equals 5 grams of olive oil, or the equivalent of one small teaspoon of olive oil. Even as large a dose as fifty capsules of Lyprinol a day is not a high-calorie fat item. In fact, this amount is minuscule compared with what we eat normally. When we eat french fries or untrimmed steak, we eat much more fat in a few mouthfuls than we'll find in an entire bottle of Lyprinol!

*Carotenoids:* The primary anti-inflammatory agents identified in Lyprinol are carotenoids. Carotene is found fairly frequently in fruits and in vegetables such as carrots and dark-leafed greens. The carotenoids are responsible for giving Lyprinol its dark orange color. Scientists are still investigating which particular carotenoids are present in Lyprinol. In fact, there has been some speculation that the carotenoids may be unique because so far they have defied exact identification. Certainly, scientists have discovered a wide range of different types of carotenoids in Lyprinol. It is possible that they are derived from the plankton that forms the steady diet of the green-lipped mussel.

What do carotenoids do in the body? They are antioxidants. That means they help protect against agents in the blood called *free radicals*. No, free radicals are not people with bizarre political philosophies who have been let out of jail. They are atoms that bond with various chemical agents, leading to damage caused by oxidation. (Think of what happens when water meets with metal, leading to oxidative rust.) Carotenoids circulate through the body, scavenging for free radicals and protecting against oxidative damage. Some carotenoids, such as beta-carotene, are converted by the body to vitamin A. However, unlike vitamin A supplements, which are toxic if taken in too-high dosages, you cannot overdose on the beta-carotene found in Lyprinol.

The practical outcomes of this protection are very important and far-reaching. For example, beta-carotene protects patients who are sensitive to sunlight. Every time you soak up the sun, you absorb rays that lead to a damaging oxidative process in your skin. Melanin, the brown pigment responsible for the golden suntan worshipped by Americans, is designed to protect against this photo damage. Too much sun, however, introduces damage beyond the protection that melanin can provide. Antioxidants quench the photo-oxidative process and shield the body from the inflammatory effects of sunburn. But don't go ahead and use Lyprinol as sunscreen. It's powerful, but not by itself enough to shield you at the beach—you need all those extra skin-protection factors in sunscreen.

Lyprinol and other antioxidants are not only useful in preventing sun-induced skin damage. Free radicals are thought to be partially responsible for skin changes associated with aging. Antioxidants such as beta-carotene may help keep those wrinkles and crow's-feet at bay!

Antioxidant protection is not only skin-deep. Major health conditions can be allayed or prevented by taking antioxidants. A recently published study of more than eighty-nine thousand female nurses from 1980 through 1989 showed that women whose diet included large quantities of vitamin A were less likely to develop breast cancer than women with low intakes of vitamin A—and remember, beta-carotene is converted to vitamin A by the body. As you will see in later chapters of this book, Lyprinol's antioxidative effects can be helpful in alleviating a variety of conditions.

# Lyprinol as a Component of Good Health

As we have seen, Lyprinol is powerful and efficacious in promoting good health. But it's not a panacea. It must be incorporated into a lifestyle that includes proper nutrition, a regular exercise regimen, and stress reduction. We will look at these important elements of a healthy lifestyle later in the book.

Now let's see how Lyprinol can address your individual health needs.

# 3

•

# Joint Disorders:
# Risks and Self-Care

Many of you have purchased this book because of the word *arthritis* on the book cover. You're seeking relief from the pain and disability associated with arthritis, and are considering Lyprinol as a viable option—with good reason. Lyprinol's track record in alleviating symptoms of arthritis is excellent. But before we can discuss the role that Lyprinol might play in helping you with your disease, we must first review what arthritis is and how it comes about. It's also important to familiarize yourself with existing self-care and treatment approaches to arthritis and other joint disorders so as to put Lyprinol's unique contribution into proper perspective. This chapter will take you on a tour of your skeletal system and what places it at risk. You'll learn what you can do to protect your joints. The next chapter will take a closer look at arthritis, explaining what it is, how it is being approached by doctors today, and how Lyprinol can be helpful.

# An Introduction to Your Joints

We've all seen skeletons. They leer at us on Halloween, they stand in the corners of biology classrooms, and they appear in horror movies. As familiar as we are with what they look like, many of us don't understand exactly what they're made of or what holds them together.

The skeleton is the body's supportive framework. It consists mostly of bone, cartilage, and connective tissue. Joints are the connections between any two pieces of skeleton. They enable us to move.

Here are the skeleton's functional divisions.

- The skull, which is primarily a protective bucket turned over the brain.

- The vertebral column, which protects the spinal cord and allows freedom of movement. Even more important, it serves as an attachment for the rib cage (the crate that protects the major internal organs), the shoulder and hip girdles, and the appendages (arms and legs) that attach to them. Each appendage (arm or leg) consists of three parts—a large bone closest to the body, one large and one small bone (or one thick and one thin bone) in the middle, and then a number of small bones in the hands or feet.

Flexibility and mobility are the two most important functions of the joints. Imagine a long, hard branch. If you want to bend it, you'd have to break it. Now imagine two branches, laid out end to end. In order to form a single unit that can bend into an L, there must be some flexible connection between the two branches. In our bodies, these are called joints.

We often take good joint health for granted. This is a mistake. The strength and resilience of your joints depend on good maintenance. Joints must be used regularly. Some of the stiffness you experience when you remain in one position for too long comes from the joint's stiffening up, due to disuse. Physical exercise keeps your joints limber. You also must maintain the strength and health of your bones through engaging in weight-bearing activities. And don't neglect your muscles. Continue to strengthen them through appropriate exercises. All three—muscles, bones, and joints—are part of a total system. For each to remain healthy, the others must also be healthy.

# Healthy Joints: What They Need in Order to Function

Healthy bones are hard. They are strong and inflexible—which means they don't bend. If you want to wiggle your finger, kneel, or wave your hand, you need flexibility at the point where your bones meet—the joint. Because the bones are hard, bending the area between them might cause them to rub against each other. This is awkward, painful, and not very efficient. Your body is supplied with *cartilage* that serves as a buffer between the bones. Healthy cartilage is moist. It is well hydrated and lubricated by *synovial fluid.* This reduces friction when bone surfaces move across each other.

Cartilage is an amazingly versatile material. It's strong, but also springy. It's flexible but won't allow your joints to be bent into destructive positions. Cartilage contains three major components: water, proteoglycans (chemicals consisting primarily of a protein core), and collagen, another agent produced by the body. Collagen is the most important component of cartilage and is responsible for maintaining its structural integrity. However, the proteoglycans are also very important. They contain additional components that are currently under investigation—including glycosaminoglycan, chondroitin sulfate, and keratin sulfate. We will return to some of these later, when we discuss approaches to arthritis.

We've looked at what joints are, and how they function when they're healthy. Now let's look at unhealthy joints. What might damage a joint? What puts it at risk? And what happens inside the joint when it is damaged?

# What Places Joints at Risk?

Arguments have abounded among scientists for centuries regarding "nature versus nurture." Are we formed primarily by inborn, genetic factors or by environmental factors? Today's scientists believe that this dichotomy is too simplistic, and that the answer to this question isn't black-and-white. Rather, a mixture of genetic and environmental factors contributes to most illness. Joint diseases are no exception. People with genetic tendencies toward joint disorders are more vulnerable to environmental insults; conversely, people who continually abuse their joints may develop injury-induced disorders, even if such conditions do not run in their families.

Let's look at risk factors for joint disorders—circumstances and conditions that raise the risk of falling victim to diseases of the joints. While we're at it, we'll suggest some solutions to minimize the potential damage.

# Genetic Factors

While scientists have not yet identified the specific genes responsible for the development of joint disorders—especially osteoarthritis (OA)—it is known that these conditions tend to run in families. If you have a family history of OA, you may develop the disorder as a result of the normal aging process, even if you protect your joints. It is likely that the first signs will appear after you turn fifty-five. If you have been involved with sports, you may develop symptoms sooner.

When I use the word *symptoms,* I don't necessarily mean excruciating pain, swelling, or inflammation. Some people have joints that are stressed and damaged, but are not inflamed. These people do not suffer from pain or great discomfort. Others have relatively minor signs of joint damage—at least based on the evidence of X rays and biopsies—but have a great deal of inflammation. These individuals suffer greatly. And many people have damage that falls between the two extremes.

If arthritis runs in your family, it imperative that you become involved in a joint-protection program as early as possible. It is likely that by the time you read this book, the important time for beginning your joint protection will already be behind you. Ideally, you should have begun to take measures to shield your joints from injury while you were in your teens. But if you're a teenager, you're probably on the ball field, at the movies, or eating pizza with your friends rather than reading a book about Lyprinol and arthritis. And, obviously, you can't turn back the clock. You *can*, however, teach your own children how to protect their joints. And at whatever stage in life you find yourself, you can begin to care for your joints now.

# Sports

Sports play a big role in the long-term progression of OA. Scientists have focused a great deal of attention on people involved in sports, and have studied the impact of athletic activities on their joints. Professional athletes, colleges students who are intensely involved in sports—especially those who are attending college courtesy of an athletic scholarship of some sort—and people who regularly engage in a sport as a hobby (say, tennis or skiing) are all vulnerable to sport-induced injuries. By "injuries" I don't necessarily mean broken arms and sprained ankles. Rather, I'm talking about a more subtle process—the damage done by years of straining the same set of joints.

For example, you may have developed a style of running—a particular set of motions you use to place one foot in front of the other. Or you may have developed an especially powerful tennis serve that knocks your opponent cold every time. Insofar as these moves "work," you feel that they are functional—you do, after all, manage to run to your destination, or hit the tennis ball into your opponent's court. And insofar as you don't limp off the track or the court with serious injuries, you also feel that you're doing no harm to yourself. But actually, you may be inflicting subtle insults upon your joints with every game. You may have learned a series of moves or techniques that stress your joints and cause long-term damage.

It's easy to disregard the notion of an injury that develops over time, a process that creeps up as you age. Most eighteen-year-olds, for example, never imagine that one day they'll be eighty. Most twenty-five-year-olds think themselves to be virtually invulnerable to the slow deteriorative process of aging. Look back to your own youth. Didn't you do a few foolish things, never believing that they would catch up with you? Athletes are particularly notorious for disregarding the wear and tear put on their body by their physical activities. Precisely because of their physical prowess, they think of themselves as being above the normal physiological processes that affect the rest of us mortals. The result: They do severe damage to their joints. I have seen thirty- and thirty-five-year-olds with crippling OA induced by irresponsible athletic activities such as the repeated use of shoes with poor support or inadequate cushioning. These patients, who should be in the prime of their physical lives, are invalids.

There is also a series of destructive beliefs that abound among athletes, many of whom are subjected to extreme peer pressure to internalize and act on those beliefs. One of the most destructive attitudes I've heard is "no pain, no gain." People have come to believe that without experiencing pain, their exercise is worthless. For some athletes, this philosophy is carried to the point of masochism. Remember that pain is an important signal. It is your body's way of informing you that something is wrong. It waves a red flag in front of your face, begging you to stop whatever activity is causing the pain. Individuals who suffer from disorders that prevent them from experiencing physical pain are not to be envied, as wonderful as a pain-free life may sound. They are vulnerable to all sorts of illness- and injury-induced complications because they lack the warning signal that informs them that an illness or injury is taking place.

Pain should be responded to not only by discontinuing the offending activity, but also by taking some type of medication that will alleviate it. As far back as the 1920s, studies showed that if the sensation of pain is stopped by injecting an anesthetic at the trunk of the affected nerve, inflammation at the end of the nerve is also prevented. The anesthetic is not in and of itself an anti-inflammatory agent. Rather, the pain seems to release inflammatory substances. By blocking the pain, you also block the release of these substances. Painkillers such as acetaminophen that are not anti-inflammatory in action nevertheless can be helpful for those suffering from arthritis because they help to break the vicious cycle of inflammation. A study published in the *New England Journal of Medicine* showed that acetaminophen is as effective as an NSAID for most people who suffer from osteoarthritis. While excessive doses can lead to liver damage, ordinary doses are free from side effects.

Joint protection can be accomplished by taking a responsible approach to sports. Always be sure you receive proper coaching and training. A good coach isn't necessarily the person who knows the best strategies to stymie the opposing football team. A good coach will know the best strategies to protect your joints from injury. This is even more important than winning the game. You will have to live with your joints long after the applause and fanfare have died down. Whether you will be able to run, walk, or even sit without pain will depend on how you handle your joints during your athletic years.

With the assistance of your trainer or coach, you can observe your exercise style. Do you run heel first or toe first? Do your feet come down on their sides? You can purchase special inserts for your athletic shoes, depending on where your feet fall when you run. These serve as shock absorbers, cushioning your feet from the repetitive blows that take place every time they meet the concrete.

Minimizing shock is very important. Obviously if you play basketball, you're likely to be pounding your feet against concrete; but if you're a runner, try to choose a soft surface like a dirt track rather than a hard concrete track. And always make sure your footwear is in good shape so as to provide maximum cushioning.

# Microtrauma

Microtraumas are tiny traumas. Each one would not be powerful enough to cause injury, but a series of these little traumas can eventually cause a great deal of damage. Imagine a rock with water dripping down on it. Each drop of water has no impact on the rock. But a steady trickle of droplets, over enough time, will erode the rock and eventually make a hole in it.

Leaping out of bed in the morning places daily stress on the joints. If you tend to oversleep, then catapult yourself into your clothes, you are not giving your joints enough time to become lubricated after a period of relative immobility during the night. Many alarm clocks come with "snooze" buttons. If you set your clock to go off a few minutes before you actually need to get up, you can get the rust out of your joints while moving slowly in bed. By the time your "snooze" has alerted you to the time when you *really* need to get up, you have begun the lubricative process and have thereby protected your joints from assault.

Your morning style isn't the only factor that can lead to progressive assaults on your joints. There are a variety of professions that involve physical activities that "drip-drip" steadily until joints have been damaged. These activities are not, in and of themselves, injurious. It is the steady and prolonged repetition that causes injury. People who stand on their feet all day, such as hairdressers, dentists, salesclerks, airline attendants, or waiters, put a great deal of weight on their hips, knees, and ankles. People who engage in repetitive activities that involve the knees or hips, or the hands, elbows, or shoulders may develop arthritis—especially if they are subjected to vibrations. Such people may work on a conveyer belt at a factory, or may be involved in repairing machinery. Certainly construction workers and others who engage in repetitive lifting and lugging of heavy objects place their joints at risk.

Here, too, you need to take careful note of your lifestyle. What do you do the most? Are you a door-to-door letter carrier? You will need shoes that support your feet in the type of walking you do. Are you a waiter who does a lot of standing (while taking orders) and then walking (to and from the kitchen)? You may need to purchase footwear that is designed for these types of activities. In Europe, for example, waiters wear special shoes. So do nurses, salesclerks, beauticians, dentists, and dental assistants. These shoes may not look as though they belong in a fashion show. In fact, they may be downright ugly. But aesthetics are far less important than health. Specialized shoe stores often have computers that help you find a shoe that fits your feet and your activities.

If you work at a computer, with your wrists immobilized for long periods of time on the keyboard, or if you work on a conveyer belt, repeatedly removing damaged items, for example, you will need to remind yourself to take frequent breaks. Some mild stretching exercises may offset some of the damaging effects of these repetitive motions. You may need to fight for your right to do this on the job, but I encourage you to use every means at your disposal to do so. Employers are becoming increasingly aware of work-induced injuries. It is in their best interests to provide the most health-enhancing work environment for their employees, so as to cut down on sick time and also to avoid legal action in the event of injury.

# Balancing Your Legs: Achieving Symmetry

It may sound strange to you, but your legs probably are not completely symmetrical. This doesn't mean that you look grotesquely lopsided, but simply that for most people, one leg is almost always just a little longer than the other. And the difference between the legs rarely remains constant because at a certain point, we stop growing. We grow until the age of twenty-five, after which we start to lose height. Rarely does this process balance out the legs. More often, it accentuates the difference. So if you want to protect your hips, spine, and knees from wear and tear induced by imbalance, it's important to balance your legs on a regular basis. An orthopedist or podiatrist can measure the distance between your heel and the crest of your iliac bone. This may sound easy, but don't try it on your own. It's important to be assessed by a professional on a regular basis because even just millimeters and fractions of millimeters have a consequence over the long term. Then you maintain the balance of your legs by inserting and wearing an appropriate inner sole.

# Other Environmental Factors

Arthritis is aggravated by cold, damp environments. The United Kingdom and Scandinavia, both of which have cold, damp climates, are known for their high rates of arthritis. If you have a family history of arthritis—and even if you don't—make sure you keep yourself warm and dry at all times. Don't lie around in your wet bathing suit. Change into dry clothes as soon as possible. Take an extra sweater or scarf wherever you go in case the weather turns unexpectedly chilly. Make sure your bedcovers are thick and cozy, and sleep in a warm room. That way if you uncover yourself during the night, you won't get chilled.

# Nutritional Factors

We already discussed nutrition in detail in chapter 2, so we won't engage in extensive repetition here. However, it is worth touching on a few of the points we made earlier, because they are so important and so easy to forget.

Remember that the strong preponderance of trans-fatty acids as well as omega-6 oils in our diet sets us up for inflammation. The omega-6 group increases the supply of arachidonic acid, the precursor of prostaglandins, thromboxanes, leukotrienes, and other mediators of inflammation. Individuals living in southern Greece, for example, have a very low incidence of rheumatoid arthritis be-

cause they eat large quantities of cooked vegetables and use primarily olive oil—a natural source of monounsaturated fatty acids
(MUFAs).

Interestingly, the French also have a lower incidence of joint
disorders. Why is that? They don't eat large quantities of fish oil,
nor are they known for their consumption of omega-3 oils, such
as olive, flaxseed, or borage. Scientists refer to this as the "French
paradox." They have come to believe that duck, goose, and chicken
fats—staples of the southwestern French diet—are actually rich in
monounsaturated fatty acids. Even butter and cream, when eaten
raw, do not necessarily have deleterious effects on the system. It is the
*heating* of these fats that causes them to become trans-fatty acids,
with all their destructive results.

If you want to protect your joints, you must begin to make some
dietary changes. These will be helpful not only for your joints but
also for your cardiovascular system, as we'll see in the next chapter.
They are recommended for everyone, and they are imperative for individuals with a family history of arthritis.

- Switch to MUFA-rich vegetable oils, such as canola and
  olive oils.

- Many animal fats that are consumed in small amounts carry
  MUFAs; foie gras, schmaltz, and raw butter are certainly
  healthier than margarine or "spreads." However, you should
  avoid organ meats, red meats, and egg yolks because they're
  high in the type of fats that store arachidonic acid.

  If you must have red meat or eggs, then use range-fed
  cattle and wild game, and eggs from free-range chickens.
  These tend to be lower in fat, and the fat they do contain is
  usually lower in arachidonic acid. Trim as much visible fat

as possible from your steaks. Try grilling rather than frying, and marinate your red meat in a mixture of 1 cup of red wine and 1 cup of olive or light sesame oil for twenty-four hours. Drain, season, and grill. The wine leaches out a fair amount of saturated fat in the steak, and the olive oil replaces it with monounsaturated fat.

Make omelets from two egg whites per one egg yolk. You can scramble your eggs with ricotta cheese or tofu to add consistency and flavor. Experiment with removing egg yolks from recipes.

- Avoid cookies, crackers, and foods processed with "hydrogenated" oils. They contain trans-fatty acids.

- Increase your consumption of fish, such as salmon, mackerel, and other seafood that is high in fat. They are high in omega-3 PUFAs. However, if you hate fish or are allergic to it, you can certainly obtain these PUFAs from vegetable oils. And, of course, you can supplement with a high-quality marine-oil supplement such as Lyprinol. We will discuss supplementation later in this chapter.

- Saturated fat shouldn't be rejected entirely. For instance, coconut and palm oils demonstrate powerful antioxidant properties that offset their potential danger as "rich in saturated fats." The key is balance.

- BALANCE your fats. Your ratio of omega-6 to omega-3 PUFAs should be 1–2:1. That means you should be eating at most twice as much omega-6 as omega-3 PUFAs. Monounsaturated fats are also acceptable.

- LIMIT your fats. A good diet should provide less than two thousand calories a day. You should keep your fat intake to less than 20 percent of your total caloric intake. And keep those trans-fatty acids to a minimum. Sure, enjoy a plate of french fries or a few "cream-in-the-middle" cookies from time to time, but be sure you keep your quantities small and your intake very occasional.

- Good nutrition doesn't only involve oils. You need a well-balanced diet with enough protein, vegetables, vitamins, and minerals. You need fiber. Processed foods are notoriously low in fiber and in important minerals, such as magnesium. Magnesium is an important mineral for those who want to prevent arthritis, or to reduce its symptoms. Good sources of magnesium include traditional hearty, solid breads; whole-wheat pasta; legumes; dried fruits; nuts; and some mineral waters.

- Remember to drink plenty of water. People who have a tendency for arthritis have even more need for water than do others. Why? Because water is an essential component of healthy cartilage. It is necessary for the lubrication of the area between the joints. While coffee, tea, alcohol, and soft drinks all provide liquid, water is best because it flushes out impurities and toxins in the joints instead of adding more.

    How much water should you drink? Divide your body weight in half. That's how many ounces of water you need to absorb each day to flush toxins out of your joints. You don't have to have it all in the form of fluids. Remember that there is water in many foods.

- Avoid chili peppers. Capsaicin, which is their active ingredient, releases a chemical called Substance P that creates inflammation around nerve endings. It will aggravate an inflammatory process if it runs in your family.

So as you can see, your diet is a crucial aspect of your overall health and is very important in helping you prevent arthritis and reduce the symptoms if you already suffer from it.

# Obesity

Obesity is not merely a cosmetic problem. It is a medical problem as well, and it has reached almost epidemic proportions in most Western countries. Being overweight puts strain and pressure on joints, even when you're lying down. After all, the horizontal position does not suppress gravity. If we were not subject to the laws of gravity even while lying down, we'd float into space at bedtime. So the pressure on our bones and joints is real, even if there is no vertical gravity involved.

When you're standing, the pressure on joints rises, because the joints must lug around heavier and heavier loads. The combination of overeating, guzzling soft drinks like soda, and living a sedentary lifestyle contribute to obesity. It has been thoroughly documented that young girls who watch too much television and eat excessively large quantities of fattening foods, for example, are more likely to be obese and to develop arthritic conditions at an early age—especially in their hips and knees, which are the joints that must carry the extra weight. Arthritis doesn't confine itself to overweight individuals, but obesity certainly increases the risk.

# Stress

Whose life doesn't contain some stress? If you're reading these words and you believe you qualify, please contact me with your secret. Most of us experience stress at one point or other in our lives. I'm not just talking about major psychological traumas—death or illness of a loved one, job loss or divorce. Even the "minor" day-to-day glitches and difficulties (schedules too tightly packed, unanticipated workload, a plumber who doesn't show up, for example) are stressful.

There is some good evidence that people who are under stress have an unconscious tendency to contract their muscles. Tension headaches, for example, are caused by the tightening up of neck muscles. Fibromyalgia is a syndrome that has been identified relatively recently. While scientists are still investigating exactly what it is, we do know that it's associated with tension in neck and back muscles that leads to pain. So psychological stress doesn't confine itself to the mind. It affects the muscles as well. Tense, contracted muscles, in turn, have a negative impact on the joints. It is harder for bones to move freely when muscles are contracted. The muscle spasm constricts the joint and, over time, can cause damage.

Techniques such as yoga, biofeedback, meditation, relaxation, and visualization that relieve psychological stress also relieve the physical stress. This, in turn, improves and reduces the inflammation associated with the underlying damage.

# Exercise

Exercise builds muscle strength and also relieves psychological stress. I'm not talking here about sports activities. Rather, I'm talking about aerobic exercise as well as strength-building exercises such as weight lifting. As with any physical activity, there is the potential of injury, so it's important to check with an exercise therapist, coach, or trainer before embarking upon an exercise program. You must make sure you are not engaging in repetitive motions that will ultimately cause more stress than they alleviate. You should also be checked over by your physician, especially if you're over the age of forty-five. It's important to have a clean bill of health before embarking on an exercise program. If you are experiencing some type of health problem, you may need specialized advice about how to exercise safely.

Having covered all the bases, get started on an exercise regimen! Safe exercise has enormous benefits for your joints as well as your psyche.

Here's an activity that might relieve both psychological and physical stress—and involves a certain amount of physical exercise and activity. I'm referring to sex. People who enjoy a happy sex life tend to have less stress and less pain. It is well documented that orgasms, especially in women, produce some analgesia that relieves pain. There can also be a great release of tension in the orgasm—not to mention the additional emotional benefits of intimacy, support, and companionship that are so important if you are going through a difficult time. I'm not suggesting that you become a nymphomaniac! Simply that you make time to incorporate this wonderful and natural stress-reducer into your life on a more frequent basis.

Now that we've looked at a variety of lifestyle issues that place joints at risk and have suggested lifestyle modifications to address them, let's turn to arthritis itself and study it more closely. What is it? What causes it? And, beyond the changes suggested above, what can be done to prevent and treat it? Are current treatment approaches effective? How can Lyprinol help?

# 4

•

# Lyprinol and
# Joint Diseases

• *George, age forty-eight, owned a garden-maintenance and landscaping business. He developed severe, rapidly progressive rheumatoid arthritis. For fourteen months, he experienced pain, stiffness, weakness of his hands and wrists, and difficulty walking. He was seriously considering giving up his landscaping business and associated garden center as he could no longer manage the work or drive his trucks. He was taking a nonsteroidal anti-inflammatory drug (NSAID) called Naproxen together with aspirin—to no avail. He was in physical pain and was also very depressed.*

*George began taking four capsules a day of Lyprinol. He did not show up for his follow-up appointment, which was scheduled for a month after his initial appointment. Later he apologized. He had been outdoors in a massive blizzard, laying a driveway for a local estate. He had been so intent on the proj-*

ect that he had simply forgotten the appointment. He reported that at first, his symptoms worsened. The hardest day was the third after beginning treatment with Lyprinol. After that, the pain and swelling subsided, his strength improved, and he was able to do all the heavy jobs associated with his business.

- Mary, age forty-one, was initially diagnosed with rheumatoid arthritis. She had begun to feel unwell approximately one year prior to being seen. She developed increasing stiffness and felt she was aging rapidly. Mary suffered from severe fatigue and pronounced weakness of the arms and hands. She woke up in the morning feeling stiff, and remained so all day. She had difficulty bending down and climbing stairs. Prior to the illness, she had been very active. One of her favorite activities had been horseback riding. For several months, she had been unable to ride. She was very despondent because she missed her horse. The ibuprofen that she was taking upset her stomach and did little to alleviate the pain and stiffness. Her saliva and tears had dried up during the course of the illness, so she was also taking artificial saliva and tears.

  Two weeks after starting Lyprinol (four capsules per day) she was feeling much better. Her stiffness and pain were gone, and her strength had returned. So had her tears and saliva. She had much more energy and had started to ride her horse again. One week later, she was riding with ease.

  She has continued to do well and has no problems with her joints, eyes, or saliva as long as she continues to take the lipid extract. When she forgets or runs out of Lyprinol, the symptoms return, but are reversed rapidly when she recommences taking the extract. She no longer needs any NSAIDs or artificial tears or saliva.

- *Bonita, age forty-three, thought she was suffering from arthritis, which ran in her family. Although the diagnosis had never been confirmed, her shoulders were often stiff and painful, especially on awakening and before a rainstorm. She also suffered from fibromyalgia and constant neck and head pain due to two herniated discs at the base of her scalp.*

  *Bonita was unable to take ibuprofen for the pain because of its negative effects on the stomach coupled with her history of ulcers. She tried using acetaminophen, but her headaches continued to worsen and began to affect her work and her relationships.*

  *Bonita heard about Lyprinol through a friend and began using it to alleviate the symptoms of arthritis. She knew that there was no risk in trying Lyprinol because it has no negative side effects. Within two weeks, the pain in her shoulders had completely disappeared. She also found, to her amazement, that many of her other symptoms had resolved. Her neck pain became almost negligible, the general fibromyalgia-induced achiness throughout her body disappeared, and she has not had a single headache since starting Lyprinol.*

George, Mary, and Bonita are examples of three people who successfully used Lyprinol to heal serious arthritis. They are not alone. Lyprinol has been demonstrated effective in relieving joint swelling and pain due to a variety of conditions. Before we can understand the unique contribution Lyprinol can make to the treatment of arthritis, we must first understand what arthritis is and how doctors currently approach it.

# An Introduction to Inflammation

Damage to joints causes inflammation to both the joints and their adjacent tissues—inflammation that leads to pain, stiffness, joint enlargement, and more inflammation.

What is inflammation anyway?

When you sustain an injury, or when an alien organism such as a virus, fungus, or bacterium invades, the body responds by releasing a series of chemicals. These chemicals can cause redness, swelling, pain, and impeded function. Strange as this may sound, these are actually desirable bodily responses, as unpleasant as they may be. They are the body's way of protecting you against infection. Injury damages the integrity of the skin or other internal surfaces, as well as connective tissue, muscle, and blood vessels. This places you at risk of infection, which can be caused by the entry of harmful organisms through the ruptured and damaged surface. The body must respond to injury by repairing and healing the damaged tissue. To do so, the blood vessels expand so as to transport more chemicals to the affected area. The tiny blood vessels—the capillaries—become more permeable. This means that the usually tight, protective blood-vessel walls relax to allow larger molecules of invasion fighters out so as to do "battle" with the invading organism, or help repair the damaged site. Finally, chemicals leave the capillaries and enter surrounding tissues.

Among the many powerful chemicals released by the capillaries are leukotrienes, which we discussed in detail in chapter 2. Remember: Leukotrienes are produced by the LOX pathway. The COX pathway releases other inflammatory substances called prostaglandins and thromboxanes. Each plays a different role in creating inflammation.

In autoimmune diseases, such as arthritis and asthma, the body reacts by calling in the equivalent of the National Guard, as if there were a foreign invader—when in reality, none is present. Of course, after our discussion of risk factors, you can understand that in reality, there is a small but steady stream of "microinvaders"—mini-insults causing minor, undetectable inflammatory responses that eventually build up over time to create a state of chronic inflammation. It is as if the soldiers "set up camp" at a particular site and never leave, because they continue to "expect" an invasion to occur.

However, there are two different types of arthritis—osteoarthritis (OA) and rheumatoid arthritis (RA). While the inflammatory process occurring in each may be similar, and microtraumas may play an important role in both conditions, osteoarthritis is more frequently caused by "impact injury" or the "wear and tear" of life. It more commonly creeps up with the onset of older age. RA, on the other hand, is strictly an autoimmune disorder. While it may be exacerbated by serious or minor injury, it is not *caused* by these factors. Ultimately, scientists are still struggling to understand why the body suddenly "decides" to turn against itself in autoimmune disorders.

Both types of arthritis seem to have their chemical origins right in the affected joints. It has been discovered that joints contain *mast cells*. These special cells play an important role in the inflammatory process. When activated, they release preformed inflammatory mediators associated with inflammation—like histamine, the leukotrienes, prostaglandins, and thromboxanes. Uncovering the role of mast cells in inflammation represents an important scientific discovery because it demonstrates that inflammation in the joints is not imported from elsewhere in the body, but originates in the joints themselves. This makes joints even more vulnerable than previously thought to the steady onslaught of microtraumas and other injuries.

# Arthritis and Inflammation

Arthritis does its damage by causing inflammation to the joints and adjacent tissues. This inflammation leads to pain, stiffness, cracking, joint enlargement, and, in turn, more inflammation. In fact, the word *arthritis* literally means "joint inflammation." It is a catchall term, however, referring to a group of more than one hundred rheumatic diseases that can cause pain, stiffness, and swelling in the joints. These diseases may affect not only the joints but also other parts of the body including important supporting structures such as muscles, bones, tendons, and ligaments, as well as some internal organs.

Some 40 to 50 million Americans—one in seven people—are said to suffer from arthritis, and almost everyone over the age of fifty has signs of it. It is estimated that by the year 2020, 60 million people in the United States will have some form of arthritis. And although arthritis can affect people in the prime of their lives (almost 9 million adults), there is a higher prevalence in elderly individuals. Women are more likely than men to suffer from arthritis. In fact, arthritis is the most prevalent chronic condition in women, affecting 22.8 million in 1990. Whether you're male or female, you are at serious risk of disability if you suffer from arthritis, which is the leading cause of disability in America. It causes limitations of activity in approximately 7 million Americans. That means it causes more disability than heart and lung conditions, diabetes, or cancer! These are disturbing and sobering figures. It is not an exaggeration to say that arthritis is a national emergency.

When you see an elderly person hobbling along, painfully leaning on a cane, you can assume the person probably is suffering from some form or arthritis. Movement is difficult, labored, and painful. The fingers move slowly, the legs no longer appear to obey the person's commands. Inflammation has run amok and is causing serious damage to mobility. As modern medicine continues to find new and exciting ways to prolong life, and the population of senior citizens continues to rise, we will see an increasing number of older adults who cannot enjoy the gift of long life to its fullest.

Let's move away from these grim statistics and predictions and look at what can be done for those who suffer from arthritis. The good news is that there's plenty to do—and that Lyprinol can play a crucial role in painting a more optimistic picture of the future.

# Types of Arthritis

We've touched briefly on the distinction between the two types of arthritis—OA and RA. While they may have some similar symptoms and, certainly, both are caused by inflammation, they have a different cause and also affect different parts of the body.

Rheumatologists—doctors who are concerned with connective-tissue diseases—look at two pairs of major joints, the knees and the hips, for the diagnosis of osteoarthritis (OA).

With gout and rheumatoid arthritis (RA), the small joints like those in the hands (and with gout, the toes) are mainly affected, although large joints can also be involved. Many more people are affected with OA because it's associated with aging and trauma; RA and gout, on the other hand, have a stronger genetic component.

Let's look at OA and RA in greater detail before turning to the role of Lyprinol in alleviating some of the destructive results of the inflammatory process.

# Osteoarthritis (OA): The Effects of Aging

OA is often called "wear and tear" arthritis because it is usually caused by the impact of a prolonged series of microtraumas associating with the normal process of daily life, rather than with an autoimmune disorder of unknown origin. There are at least twenty-five different forms of OA. Although it can occur in people under the age of forty-five, it most often occurs with the onset of age. It is a slow and progressive condition that generally affects the weight-bearing joints of the knees and hips, as well as the lower back, neck, and fingers.

While the inflammation in OA comes from several different locations in and around the bone, cartilage breakdown is its main feature. Inflammatory mediators are increased in the damaged cartilage. Additionally, surrounding fluid—called *synovial* fluid—also exudes some inflammatory substances. These are called matrix metalloproteinases, collagenases, and prostaglandins. Together with other chemical agents, these degrade the collagen and proteoglycans present in healthy cartilage. Nitrous oxide production increases, and a process called *apoptosis* occurs. Apoptosis means "programmed cell death." It happens when cells self-destruct because they have become too damaged to survive and to replicate into new, healthy cells. As OA progresses, more cartilage is degraded, and the mechanics of joint use change. These joint changes create additional irritation, which further promotes inflammation; and so the process continues and the condition worsens.

As mentioned, OA is not a single condition. It can take many different forms. For example, *chondritis* occurs when chondrocytes—the cartilage cells responsible for producing building blocks of

healthy cartilage—synthesize prostaglandins, which are inflammatory chemicals. Chondrocytes do this in response to these *cytokines,*
which are messenger proteins that enable cells to influence one another. Cytokines are not by any means undesirable substances. On
the contrary, they are an important aspect of the body's immune system. However, in osteoarthritis, they are "overmessaging" and "calling in the troops" inappropriately. This leads to further joint damage
and inflammation.

*Osteitis* occurs when the damage spreads to the bone, and *synovitis* occurs when the synovial lining tissue—the membrane located on
the interface between the cartilage and the bone—becomes inflamed. Synovitis occurs frequently with OA, and the degree of inflammation predicts response to nonsteroidal anti-inflammatory
drugs (NSAIDs).

The conventional medical treatments for arthritis have largely involved analgesics and NSAIDs. These are used to control the symptoms of arthritis, including pain and stiffness. Some of these
compounds are prescription drugs, while others can be obtained over
the counter. As mentioned, the principal drawback of these drugs is
their tendency to ulcerate the mucous membranes of the stomach
and intestinal tract. Some 25 percent of patients experience serious
side effects, ranging from bleeding ulcers, to stomach and intestinal
discomfort, to liver and kidney problems, and even death.

# Rheumatoid Arthritis (RA)

RA, which is an autoimmune disorder, is a crippling disease that affects about 2.1 million Americans, or about 1 percent of the popula-

tion—most of them women. While RA is not itself fatal, sufferers are at increased risk for other illnesses, such as adult-onset diabetes and gastrointestinal bleeding. These illnesses shorten life spans by an average of between five and fifteen years.

There are at least ninety different forms of RA whose causes are not fully understood. It can be triggered by environmental factors, a bacterial or viral infection, stress, and even hormonal imbalances following pregnancy. Although it is aggravated by injury, RA is ultimately due to a mysterious disease process that is probably genetic in origin. While a competent rheumatologist should make the diagnosis, you can guess at which condition you have based on your symptoms. RA generally is characterized by symmetrical joint swelling. That means that corresponding joints on either side of the body are likely to be affected. You may experience pain and swelling in the second and third knuckles and middle joints of both hands, for example. The balls of your toes may become painful. You may experience extended stiffness upon awakening in the morning.

Your doctor will look for swelling and thickening in the synovial lining—the lining of the joints. He or she may order laboratory tests to ascertain whether your blood shows elevated markers of inflammation. Over 75 percent of patients with RA test positive for something called *rheumatoid factor* in the blood. Your doctor may also order X rays to ascertain whether there is evidence of a narrowing in the joint space.

RA can spread to internal organs. The inflammation can move to the internal lining of the lungs (a condition called pleurisy), or to the peripheral nerves. When this happens, you may experience numbness or tingling from neuropathy. You need to be on the alert for anemia, because RA can affect the bone marrow, which is an important component of the processing of red blood cells. Your eyes and even the lining of your heart may be affected. So if you have RA, it's vital to place yourself under the care of a rheumatologist who will take regular blood tests to measure your levels of rheumatoid factor. These will provide important clues as to your vulnerability to the spread of inflammation.

# Treatment Options for Arthritis

Throughout this chapter and in the previous chapter, we have alluded to different existing treatment approaches to arthritis. It's time for a more thorough review of available treatments. Some offer short-term relief, while others boast longer-term results.

### *Painkillers*

There are several different categories of painkillers. Each works somewhat differently in the body, each has its own set of properties, and each has its own set of side effects. NSAIDs like aspirin and ibuprofen, for example, are both painkillers with anti-inflammatory benefits as well. Unfortunately, they also have serious side effects—in particular, digestive disturbances, such as gastritis, esophagitis, and bleeding ulcers. Some people develop even more serious problems, such as kidney failure, or hemorrhage in the brain. While these medications can in all fairness be considered miracle drugs because they help millions of people to experience relief from relentless pain, their side effects have been extremely problematic.

Acetaminophen is an effective painkiller, although it does not have anti-inflammatory properties. However, when used over an extended period of time, it can have a negative impact on the liver.

You can use NSAIDs and acetaminophen to obtain short-term

relief when you have a flare-up of arthritic symptoms. However, for more chronic problems, you need to look for other solutions because of the side effects associated with long-term use.

## Corticosteroids

These hormones, taken by mouth or given by injection, are very effective in treating arthritis. Prednisone is the corticosteroid most often used orally to reduce the inflammation associated with RA. The doctor might inject a corticosteroid directly into a joint to stop pain. However, frequent injections may damage the cartilage and should only be used once or twice a year. Moreover, oral steroids have an array of severe side effects.

## Surgery

Two types of surgery are used to address arthritis—palliative surgery, which is designed to alleviate pain, and replacement surgery, which replaces damaged joints with artificial alternatives. The surgeon may remove the synovium, realign the joint, or even replace the damaged joint with an artificial one. Total joint replacement has provided not only dramatic relief from pain, but also improvement in motion.

## COX-2 Inhibitors

Remember the COX pathway discussed in the previous chapter? COX-2 inhibitors such as Vioxx® and Celebrex®, which have been recently approved by the Food and Drug Administration (FDA), are supposed to work only on the COX-2 pathway. That's the one responsible for inflammation. They are supposed to leave the COX-1 pathway intact (the one responsible for maintenance of a healthy digestive tract). While they have fewer gastric side effects, they continue to exercise an adverse impact on blood vessels, kidneys, and other tissues and organs. Moreover, they are not always effective in the long run.

## Cyclosporin

A potent suppressor of the immune system, this treatment may be indicated in severe cases that are either life threatening, or completely crippling. Because suppressing the immune system can have such serious side effects, Cyclosporin should be used as a last-resort approach.

## Rub-on-Balms

Some topical ointments offer relief without systemic side effects. These include Ben Gay®, Aspercreme®, Myoflex®, Mineral Ice®, Icy Hot®, Absorbine Jr.®, Mentholatum®, Heet®, Zeel®, and Traumeel®. They cause the blood vessels to expand, and the area to feel warm, bringing relief. Usually, however, the relief is short-lived and quite local. The very advantage of a topical ointment—that it doesn't enter the system—is also its disadvantage, because its beneficial effects don't go beyond the confines of the immediate area.

## Heat and Cold

Moist heat (such as a warm bath or shower) or dry heat (such as a heating pad) placed on the painful area of the joint for about fifteen minutes may relieve the pain. An ice pack (or a bag of frozen vegetables) wrapped in a towel and placed on the sore area for about fifteen minutes may help to reduce swelling and stop the pain. (Do not use cold packs if you have poor circulation.)

## *Joint Protection*

Using a splint or a brace to allow joints to rest and protect them from injury can be helpful.

## *Massage*

Lightly stroking and/or kneading the painful muscle may increase blood flow and bring warmth to an affected area. However, because arthritis-stressed joints are very sensitive, you need to find a massage therapist with experience in dealing with arthritic patients. An inexperienced masseur or masseuse might cause further injury to the joint.

## *Acupuncture*

In acupuncture, a medical approach that originated in China, thin needles are inserted at specific points in the body. The National Institutes of Health (NIH) has endorsed the use of acupuncture for pain relief. Scientists think that application of the needles at appropriate points may stimulate the release of natural, pain-relieving chemicals produced by the brain or the nervous system.

The United States now has an accreditation procedure for acupuncturists. Make sure that the one you consult has proper qualifications. It would be helpful if he or she also has experience dealing with arthritis and other inflammatory conditions.

## *Weight Reduction*

Excess pounds put extra stress on weight-bearing joints such as the knees or hips. Studies have shown that overweight women who lost an average of eleven pounds substantially reduced the development of OA in their knees. In addition, if OA has already affected one knee, you can protect the other knee by removing weight-induced stress.

## Disease-Modifying Antirheumatic Drugs

These drugs are used to treat people with RA who have not responded to NSAIDs. Some of these include methotrexate, hydroxychloroquine, penicillamine, and gold injections. Recently monoclonal antibodies have been studied, and some have received FDA approval. These drugs are thought to influence and correct abnormalities of the immune system responsible for a disease like RA. Treatment with these medications requires careful monitoring by a physician to avoid side effects.

## Exercise

Swimming, walking, low-impact aerobic exercise, and range-of-motion exercises may reduce joint pain and stiffness. In addition, stretching exercises such as yoga are helpful.

## Glucosamine (with or without Chondroitin Sulfate)

Glucosamine is a chondro-protective agent. This means that it provides the body with the raw materials to regenerate cartilage necessary for healthy joint function.

In order for OA to be treated effectively, the cartilage and synovial fluid in the joint must be protected against further destruction. At the same time, it is desirable to stimulate restoration of joint cartilage and synovial fluid. Research seems to indicate that chondroprotective agents protect and restore joint cartilage by:

- supporting and enhancing chondrocyte synthesis
- supporting or enhancing the synthesis of synovial fluid, which is required to lubricate the joint
- inhibiting free radical enzymes and autoimmune processes that degrade joint cartilage
- removing blockages in blood vessels leading to the joint

A glucosamine deficiency caused by faulty diet, trauma, and aging contributes to the development of osteoarthritis. Nine European studies showed that the oral administration of glucosamine produced major reductions in joint pain, joint tenderness, and swelling. Improvements in joint function and overall physical performance were noted, compared with placebo and/or ibuprofen. While ibuprofen worked more rapidly than glucosamine in relieving pain, glucosamine had more long-lasting results because it became incorporated into the joint cartilage matrix, resulting in healthier cartilage and less damage to the joints. However, although glucosamine is highly promising, recent research shows that it may not be entirely free of side effects that might effect the muscles, nervous system, or kidneys.

## Other Chondro-Protective Agents

Welcome to the often-bewildering world of neutraceuticals. These are nonprescription nutritional supplements that are purported to be helpful in alleviating illnesses—in this case, arthritis. I say "bewildering" because many of these remedies have been popularized through hearsay, folk wisdom, or anecdotal evidence. There may be some truth to the contention that they work, but I can't vouch for them with any certainty. The most reliable evidence is obtained through the scientific "gold standard" of clinical studies—which are often notably absent. I am listing these remedies here for the sake of completeness. Since they are reputed to be helpful, and do not appear to do any harm, they may be worth trying.

It is important to recognize that the kind of people who are motivated enough to start taking nutritional supplements usually do not begin taking these supplements in a vacuum. Taking nutritional supplements is often accompanied by other lifestyle changes, such as the elimination of unhealthful foods from the diet, the incorporation of regular exercise into the schedule, and the adoption of stress-reduction techniques.

Dietary and health supplements from natural sources include:

- MSM (Methyl-Sulfonyl-Methane)—a natural form of sulfur found in many fresh foods including most fresh fruits and vegetables, milk, and some grains. Even though MSM is present in fresh foods, it is easily destroyed in cooking, storing, and processing, and sufficient MSM levels may not be present to provide significant biological sulfur. MSM should be used for cartilage repair and joint lubrication in OA only.
- Ginger—raw, candied, or cooked ginger seems to help people with OA. Ginger supplements are also available at health food stores.
- Multivitamin and mineral supplements, including vitamins C, E, the B group (especially B6, B12, and B3), A, and D. Mineral supplements include magnesium, calcium, zinc, and iron.
- Piasclédine®—a drug that is used in parts of Europe—is an interesting extract from soybean and avocado. A limited number of reliable studies have shown that it brought about some improvement in mild to moderate arthritis symptoms after a few months. Patients receiving placebo did not experience similar improvement. However, it had less impact on patients with severe symptoms.

- Fish oils such as Max-EPA, cod-liver oil, mussel powder (Seatone), and mussel lipids (Lyprinol)—we'll return to Lyprinol later.

### Additional Treatments

Other treatments for arthritis include hydrotherapy, heat massage, cold massage, ultrasound (deep heat), hot wax (heat therapy), other forms of massage, traction, transcutaneous electrical nerve stimulation (TENS), biofeedback, psychological counseling, and meditation.

Each of these approaches offers some hope and may represent a partial solution to the arthritis problem. It is the contention of this book, however, that over and above healthful lifestyle changes, Lyprinol is the most effective and also the safest neutraceutical supplement. It's also more effective and safer than pharmaceutical medications. The next section will look at Lyprinol and arthritis in greater detail.

# Lyprinol and Arthritis

Although OA and RA are caused by different disease processes, they have much in common. Both respond well to fish oils in general, and Lyprinol in particular. Remember that Lyprinol affects two different pathways—LOX and COX—responsible for inflammation. Remember, too, that it manages to do this without causing any of the adverse effects associated with existing antiarthritis medications, such as NSAIDs.

Let's take a closer look at some of the studies that support the beneficial impact of Lyprinol on arthritis.

- After more than twenty years of research, clinical trials have shown Lyprinol to be more effective in reducing arthritic pain and inflammation than other remedies. Additional clinical trials have demonstrated that Lyprinol can outperform proprietary pharmaceutical NSAIDs as well as remedies such as the traditional fish and plant oils containing omega-3 and omega-6 fatty acids.

- French doctors B. Audeval and P. Bouchacourt conducted a six-month randomized study of the effects of Seatone powder on OA of the knee. Of fifty-three patients, twenty-seven received stabilized Seatone every day and twenty-six received a placebo. Neither group knew whether they were receiving the real treatment or the placebo. Patients' symptoms were measured at the beginning and end of the study, and at one-month intervals during the study.

  For the first five months, neither group of patients showed any change in symptoms. Then, toward the end of the study, patients with mild to moderate forms of OA experienced symptom relief. Those with more serious symptoms experience no change, even after six months. The results, though modest, did hold promise because none of those taking the placebo improved at all.

- An ongoing study of thirteen patients with long-standing OA is currently under way in Denmark. Twelve of thirteen patients so far have reported a dramatic 50 percent reduction of pain, and 50 percent improvement in several indices of arthritis symptoms at day twenty-one through twenty-eight; the same results were confirmed at day forty-two through fifty-six. There was no increase in the use of pain relievers, and there were no side effects, including no gastric pain.

- In 2000, Dr. M. Whitehouse compared Celebrex and Vioxx, two COX-2 inhibitors, with Lyprinol and also with Anaprox®, a COX-1 inhibitor in clinical use since 1972 in laboratory rats. At a dosage rate of 15 mg/kg of body weight/day, Celebrex and Lyprinol protected against experimentally induced arthritic inflammation in the rats about equally (78 percent reduction in inflammation). Vioxx did not reduce inflammation until the dosage was raised significantly, and then it reduced inflammation only minimally. Anaprox appeared to score well. It reduced inflammation by over 80 percent. However, it also created the largest number of gastric side effects, scoring twenty-nine on the gastrotoxic scale. The other agents scored zero.

   Dr. Whitehouse concluded that Lyprinol was as effective as Celebrex, and had no adverse side effects.

- A freeze-dried powdered preparation of whole green-lipped mussels from New Zealand given orally to rats showed some modest anti-inflammatory activity. More important, it strikingly reduced the incidence of stomach ulcers in rats who were taking other NSAIDs such as aspirin and indomethacin. This implies that not only is Lyprinol free of negative side effects, but that it may actually protect against side effects induced by other medications.

- Studies carried out by Dr. Whitehouse comparing the effectiveness of Lyprinol with that of the prescription drug indomethacin showed that with a dosage of 5 mg/kg of body weight, Lyprinol was 97 percent effective in reducing swelling. In comparison, indomethacin, which is toxic at this dosage, was only 83 percent effective.

- Dr. Whitehouse and his colleagues recently compared Lyprinol to forty over-the-counter remedies, including three NSAIDs, and found it to be superior to all of them.

- Drs. Robin and Sheila Gibson conducted a clinical trial at Glasgow's Homeopathic Hospital in Scotland in the late 1970s. They used capsules of the unstabilized mussel powder—the only extract of green-lipped mussel available at that time. The Gibsons studied severely arthritic patients. They found that about a third of patients experienced considerable improvement and another third were helped to a lesser degree, although most experienced no improvement for the first three to four weeks. Even though the extract was not stabilized at that time, it was found to be safe and well tolerated. The researchers concluded that the powdered mussel was a safe and effective nutritional supplement for patients suffering from arthritis.

- In 1980, research groups from the Homeopathic Hospital and the Department of Surgery, Victoria Infirmary, Glasgow, Scotland, reported on a double-blind study involving sixty-six outpatients, twenty-eight with RA and thirty-eight with OA. All had failed to respond to conventional treatments, and all had been scheduled for surgery to improve their joint conditions.

  These patients were randomly divided into two groups. For three months, group one received the powdered mussel (still unstabilized) and group two received a placebo (dried fish-meal powder). Evaluations were done at day ninety. Then all patients were given the powdered mussel extract for three additional months. At the end of that period, results showed that 68 percent of RA and 39 percent of OA patients experienced improvement. No side effects were attributed to the mussel powder. Again, the authors concluded that the powdered mussel is an effective supplement or possible alternative to other therapies in the treatment of both RA and OA. It reduced the amount of pain and stiffness, improved the patients' ability to cope with life, and apparently enhanced general health.

• The Gibsons continued to explore the effectiveness of the New Zealand green-lipped mussel and when Lyprinol became available, they began a study comparing Seatone powder to Lyprinol. In 1998, they published their results.

There were sixty patients in the study comparing Seatone powder with Lyprinol—thirty with RA and thirty with OA. The patients in each category were randomly assigned to receive either Lyprinol or the stabilized Seatone. All previous therapy was left unaltered and no other treatment was given throughout the six months of the trial.

This approach was identical to that used in the original trial. The double-blind section of the trial was continued for three months, after which all patients were given Lyprinol for a further three months. After the final three months, all patients were assessed. The assessing physician did not know which therapy each participant had received.

The results were impressive: 76 percent of RA and 70 percent of OA patients benefited. Again the investigators concluded that Lyprinol is effective in reducing pain, swelling, and stiffness, and in improving function.

• In Denmark—another cold, damp climate—about 10 percent of the population age twenty-four to seventy-four has acute OA symptoms. Dr. Niels H. P. Hertz of Holbaek, Denmark, conducted a pilot study of the effects of Lyprinol on OA. Thirteen patients with long-standing OA in one or both knees and/or hips were included. Of the thirteen patients, twelve reported less pain at the first evaluation three to four weeks after commencement of the treatment. This result was maintained at the second evaluation.

As expected, the pain relief was accompanied by a considerable improvement in functional ability. Only one patient who completed the trial reported no significant functional improvement. Dr. Hertz concluded that Lyprinol seems to be an exceedingly potent drug against pain from OA.

# Other Rheumatological Conditions

A number of other conditions mimic or include the inflammatory effects of RA and OA. Two that we know have responded to treatment by Lyprinol are gout and ankylosing spondylitis. Let's look at them.

### Gout

Gout, which has been called the "disease of kings and the king of diseases," has been known, defined, and studied since the days of Hippocrates. Formerly a leading cause of painful and disabling chronic arthritis, gout has been all but conquered by effective treatments. Unfortunately, this information has been slow to spread to physicians and patients.

Gout, which affects an estimated 840 out of every 100,000 people, is a type of arthritis caused by an excess of uric acid in the body. People who have gout either produce too much uric acid, or they cannot properly eliminate it from their bodies. While Lyprinol is very helpful in treating gout and has been approved as a treatment for gout by the Australian government, it will be far more effective if it is used in conjunction with prescription medication. Always check with your health-care provider before combining any medications.

## Ankylosing Spondylitis

This inflammatory condition affects the spine by fusing the vertebrae together. It is very serious and can even be life threatening. Current anti-inflammatory drugs have only limited effectiveness and have serious side effects. While controlled studies have been unconvincing to date, anecdotal evidence suggests that Lyprinol may be effective in reducing inflammatory symptoms of this devastating disease. One patient, herself a physician, was unable to use the standard pharmaceutical medication (indomethacin) because of serious side effects. She began taking Lyprinol and now reports being symptom-free. Further studies are needed to replicate this extraordinary case history.

Joint disorders are just one category of illness that responds well to Lyprinol. In the next chapter, we will look at cardiovascular disease and how Lyprinol can both prevent and heal it.

# 5

•

# Lyprinol and the Heart

Here are some disturbing statistics:

- Every 29 seconds, an American will suffer a heart attack.
- Every minute, an American will die from a heart attack.
- Every 53 seconds, an American will have a stroke.
- Every 3.3 minutes, an American will die of a stroke.
- Every year about six hundred thousand Americans suffer strokes.
- One in five Americans has heart disease, stroke, or another form of cardiovascular disease. Eliminating all forms of cardiovascular disease would raise life expectancy in the United States by almost seven years.
- Cardiovascular diseases are expected to cost the U.S. an estimated $327 billion in 2001.
- Heart disease is the leading cause of disability in the U.S.

labor force, accounting for 19 percent of Social Security disability payments.
- Close to one in two women dies from cardiovascular disease.
- An estimated 22 percent of the 4,400,000 stroke survivors are permanently disabled.

The most disturbing aspect of these statistics is that *they are not necessary!* Cardiovascular disease is preventable. It is brought on by many of the unhealthy lifestyle factors we discussed in chapter 3 in connection with joint disorders, including a diet too rich in trans-fatty acids, excessive consumption of omega-6 fatty acids unbalanced by the omega-3 group, and a sedentary and high-stress lifestyle.

All these overtax the cardiovascular system. A high intake of omega-6 fatty acids makes the blood thicker and more "gluey" in consistency. The blood moves slowly through the vessels, rather than efficiently. It is more likely to get "gummed up" along the way, leading to dangerous blood clots. The extra fat builds a lining of plaque along the walls of the blood vessels. This makes them less elastic and also more narrow, so the blood has additional trouble passing through. The condition of plaque buildup along artery walls is called atherosclerosis, and is largely responsible for cardiovascular disease—especially stroke and heart attack—in Western countries.

# Omega-3 Oils in General, and Fish Oil in Particular

Incorporating more omega-3 fatty acids into the diet reduces the negative impact of the omega-6 and the trans-fatty acids. Scientists are not entirely sure whether this apparent protection is directly related to the capacity of omega-3 fatty acids to dilute viscous blood and prevent atherosclerosis, or whether it is mediated through some other means not directly related to fat metabolism. A great deal of interesting research is under way on the subject. Inflammation and atherosclerosis share similar biochemical mechanisms—at least in their early phases. This commonality has given rise to some fruitful avenues of research into the mechanism of atherosclerosis and its prevention.

It appears that the omega-3 PUFAs modify the lipid (fat) content in the blood. They increase concentrations of HDL-2, the "good" cholesterol. They also increase the levels of "good" triglyceride-rich concentration of lipoprotein (proteins bonded to fats), but keep levels of undesirable cholesterol and triglycerides down. The excessive amount of blood fat often present after a heavy meal (postprandial lipemia) can be reduced by omega-3 PUFAs—although it may sound strange to use a fat to combat another fat.

Additional benefits of fish oils include improvements in the walls of the arteries. The endothelium—the lining along the blood-vessel walls—functions more effectively. Moreover, it helps the arteries become more elastic. This flexibility is important because it allows blood to flow more rapidly and efficiently. How does it promote elasticity? By preventing the accumulation of atherosclerotic plaque.

This, in turn, is accomplished by inhibiting the growth of the cells that form the plaque.

Combating atherosclerosis is just one of many functions performed by marine-based omega-3 fats. Fish oils reduce the risk of thrombosis. Remember eicosapentaenoic acid (EPA)—an anti-inflammatory product of the omega-3 group? We explained how it prevents thrombosis by inhibiting the synthesis of thromboxane A$_2$, the prostaglandin that causes blood clotting and vascular constriction. Even if fish oil made no other contribution to human health beyond reducing the incidence of thrombosis, we'd be dealing with an invaluable substance. But fish oil does so much more. It inhibits the synthesis of LDL ("bad") cholesterol. It even has a mild blood pressure–lowering effect in both normal and mildly hypertensive individuals.

As you can see, fish oil has all kinds of benefits for the circulatory system. But these beneficial actions are not confined to the blood vessels. The EPA and DHA of fish oils have been shown to correct *ventricular fibrillation* in the heart. The ventricles are two of the heart's four chambers. Under normal circumstances, they beat in a rhythmic and methodical way. Ventricular fibrillation is a very rapid, uncoordinated series of fluttering contractions of the heart's ventricles. The heartbeat and pulse beat are no longer functioning in synchrony—a dangerous situation that can lead to heart attack.

As you can see from this summary, fish oils emerge as powerful and highly effective substances with a wide range of preventive and curative cardiovascular benefits.

# Fish Oils in General and Lyprinol in Particular

Most of studies that show EPA and DHA to be effective in addressing cardiovascular disease were carried out using an array of fish oils other than Lyprinol, but their findings also apply to the efficacy of Lyprinol. As we saw in chapter 2, very small quantities of Lyprinol are often more potent than very large quantities of fish oil. It's fair to say that any study confirming the effectiveness of fish oil can be applied to Lyprinol. It can even be assumed that Lyprinol will heighten and magnify the effect of the oil under study, since it's so much more concentrated and contains so many different types of PUFAs.

Although this is a fair assumption, studies *have* been performed to investigate whether Lyprinol is actually more effective than other fish oils. For example, one researcher named Steven Hooper compared the effectiveness of two marine oils—Fishaphos® (a commercial fish oil sold in Australia) and Lyprinol. Lyprinol slightly lowered both total and LDL cholesterol and reduced blood pressure, while the other fish oil increased both.

# Lyprinol Is Not a Blood Thinner

"You can't be too rich or too thin" the saying goes. Where blood is concerned, that's not entirely true. Although we don't want blood to be thick and gluey, we also don't want it to be too thin. It needs a certain amount of clotting factor, or you will bleed too easily; and when you bleed, you won't be able to stop quickly enough. Steven Hooper's studies showed that Fishaphos increased the risk of excessive bleeding, while Lyprinol had no effect on clotting—which means that Lyprinol remains safe even when taken together with aspirin or other blood-thinning medications, such as Coumadin (warfarin).

Why is Lyprinol so effective without some of the more problematic side effects associated with aspirin, Coumadin, and even other fish oils? Perhaps it's because Lyprinol does not affect a particular group of clotting factors, such as *prothrombin,* that are made in the liver. Its action appears to work on the level of thromboxane, another clotting factor, which is manufactured via the COX-2 pathway. Because Lyprinol does not disturb some of the major clotting factors that originate in the liver but still works against other clotting factors, it protects and maintains the ability of the blood to clot appropriately when injury is sustained.

# Lyprinol as Part of a Heart-Friendly Lifestyle

Lyprinol is not a panacea and will not fully offset the negative impact of a destructive lifestyle. Rather, it should be incorporated into an overall program to enhance your cardiovascular system. That includes the dietary changes we discussed in the previous chapter. While they were recommended in connection with preserving the health of your joints, they will also preserve the health of your heart.

Exercise is also crucial. It keeps the blood vessels toned and the circulation brisk, so that oxygen is transported to your organs more efficiently. It also helps to keep blood fat levels low.

Stress does great damage to the heart. The mechanism through which this happens is called the "fight or flight response." This phrase refers to an ancient, primeval defense mechanism programmed into our body. It's a mechanism that kicks in when we feel threatened. It appears to have originated in the bodies of our primitive ancestors who had to confront physical danger on a regular basis. When they were about to be attacked by some predatory beast, their adrenaline rose. In response, their heartbeat sped up and blood went racing through their bodies, feeding oxygen to muscles and priming them to spring into action—either to fight the beast or to flee from it. Both courses of action required massive physical expenditure, and the body responded by pumping out maximum energy.

In today's society, we are rarely attacked by raging beasts (at least four-legged ones). Our "beasts" are more likely to be nasty co-workers, uncooperative teenagers, or unpaid bills. But our primitive defense system doesn't know that. We react to these "threats" posed by our civilized society with all the same physiological ammunition that we would apply to our hypothetical jungle beast. Our heartbeat speeds up. Our palms sweat. We want to slug someone—or to run away as fast as we can. And because we live in such a stressful world, we are subjected to these "fight or flight" triggers many times a day. The strain this puts on the heart and circulatory system is enormous.

So stress-reduction techniques will help not only your joints, but also your heart. Harvard cardiologist Herbert Benson suggested meditation in his book *The Relaxation Response.* He suggested that the way to counterbalance the fight-or-flight response is to create a relaxation response. Counseling might also be a helpful way to look at the sources of stress in your life and examine how you might change them, or regard them in a different light if they cannot be changed.

The joints and the heart are not the only parts of the body to benefit from Lyprinol. The lungs will also benefit from this remarkable oil. The next chapter looks at how Lyprinol can help prevent or even cure asthma and allergies.

# 6

•

# Asthma and Allergies

- *Dimitri, age thirty-five, is a respiratory therapist. He suffered from exercise-induced asthma—especially in cold weather. If he ran or climbed stairs, for example, he began to cough and wheeze. His symptoms did not clear up until he rested and took his "rescue" remedy—one to three puffs of albuterol. He experienced episodes of wheezing that woke him up during the night. His peak expiratory flow—a standard measure of the ability of an asthmatic person to exhale—was 15 percent below normal.*

  *Dimitri also suffered from skin problems. These began with atopic dermatitis (infantile eczema), which lasted from babyhood until age eight, and even once the most severe symptoms abated, his skin remained dry and brittle. His nose was always congested, and he suffered from night thirst and loud snoring. Severe allergies run in his family—his mother and sister both suffer from asthma.*

*Eight months after starting treatment with Lyprinol, Dimitri experienced notable improvements. He has been able to reduce his use of "rescue" inhalers from two to one canister of medication per month. He has stopped snoring—a sign of less nighttime obstruction of the airways. Best of all, his peak expiratory flow is normal!*

- *Terje, age thirty-eight, is a product manager of a neutraceutical company. He suffered from severe allergic rhinitis since age twelve. During the spring season, his nose became stuffed. Beginning with March, Terje would sneeze, rub his eyes, and clear his throat. As the season progressed, he also developed exercise-induced asthma, coughing and wheezing if he attempted to run or walk. The allergy also affected his vision. Between March and June, Terje was unable to wear his contact lenses. He experienced some mild relief when he used a blue pollen mask, designed to reduce the amount of pollen he inhaled—but he hated the mask. It was uncomfortable and unsightly.*

  *Terje tried to control his symptoms by using antihistamine therapy. But the medication made him very drowsy—a serious problem, since Terje, a former air force pilot, often must fly a plane for his company. Topical corticosteroids caused his nose to start hemorrhaging, and allergy shots actually made him collapse. Injected corticosteroids had a devastating impact on his moods, precipitating a psychotic episode.*

  *Terje started taking four capsules of Lyprinol a day in February—one month before the spring symptoms usually hit. He was amazed by the result. He reported that his symptoms were about 80 percent improved. He could wear his contact lenses, drive a vehicle, pilot an airplane, and even enjoy a beer without adverse effects such as drowsiness. Best of all, he was able to hang the blue pollen mask on the wall! Terje discontin-*

*ued taking Lyprinol in June but will continue using it every spring.*

- *Gloria, age sixteen, suffered from serious asthma. She had always been prone to allergies and had experienced her first major attack of food-induced hives as an infant. At age four, she developed asthma, which continued throughout her childhood and adolescence. She needed to use her beta-antagonist inhaler many times each day and woke up wheezing at least once every night. When the inhaler was ineffective, her parents assisted her in using a nebulizer—a machine that delivers medicine to the lungs via mist. Even with the home-based nebulizer, she experienced periodic uncontrollable asthma attacks that required trips to the emergency room.*

  *Gloria began taking corticosteroids at age 10. They curtailed the asthma attacks somewhat, but caused yeast infections and weight gain that finally forced her to discontinue use after five years.*

  *For much of the time, Gloria was irritable, tense, and volatile. She was constantly tired due to interrupted sleep and also to the side effects of her medications.*

  *When she began taking Lyprinol, Gloria noticed an immediate reduction in her asthma symptoms. Within a matter of days, she stopped waking up during the night. After a week, she needed her inhaler only once a day. Her mood began to improve and her family noticed that she had become much easier to live with. One month later, Gloria is thriving, and we are hopeful that her progress will continue.*

Dimitri, Terje, and Gloria are examples of individuals who suffered from asthma and who experienced encouraging reduction of symptoms after starting Lyprinol. They are examples of millions of people worldwide who suffer from asthma, which is one of the most common chronic diseases. In all three cases, the asthma was allergic in nature and was one of several manifestations of allergy—which is a typical profile of asthmatic individuals.

Although asthma affects people of all ages, its incidence is increasing in children at an alarming rate. It occurs in all countries regardless of the level of economic development but appears to be slightly more common in poor and minority populations than among affluent Caucasians.

In the United States, asthma affects an estimated seventeen million Americans—more than 6 percent of the population—including nearly 5 million children. The disease is responsible for more than fourteen million outpatient visits to health-care professionals, nearly half a million hospitalizations, more than one million emergency room visits, and more than five thousand deaths annually. Costs associated with asthma are staggering. The disorder costs the country approximately $6.2 billion per year including both direct medical costs ($3.6 billion) and indirect costs resulting from reduced productivity, such as missed days at work or school ($2.6 billion). These grim circumstances persist despite our progress in understanding asthma and its underlying inflammatory component.

# What Is Asthma?

Asthma is a chronic disorder of the airways within the lungs and/or leading to the lungs. As these airways become inflamed, they thicken. This makes them less elastic and also more narrow. The result is that airflow to the lungs is limited. Over time, as the asthma worsens, the situation becomes exacerbated. These exacerbations can be severe and can result in death unless effective treatment is initiated.

But what exactly is asthma? Asthma has recently been redefined by the National Heart, Lung, and Blood Institute (NHLBI) as "a chronic inflammatory disorder of the airways in which many cells and cellular elements play a role, in particular, mast cells, eosinophils, T-lymphocytes, neutrophils, and epithelial cells." By now, some of these names should be familiar to you. For example, you encountered mast cells in our discussion on joints. They are cells within the cartilage that release anti-inflammatory chemicals. Epithelial cells reside along the lining of internal body cavities, such as the airways leading to the lungs. Other cells, such as eosinophils, did not pop up in any of our earlier discussions. They are usually present when some allergic process is taking place in the body. We will return to them below.

Although asthma involves inflammation of the airways leading to the lungs, it also involves chronic inflammation within the lungs themselves. When that happens, the patient develops respiratory symptoms, such as overreactivity of the airways and airflow limitation. The *bronchi* narrow and become constricted, the airway walls swell and change shape (this is called "remodeling"), and the airways become blocked by mucus plugs.

The concept of asthma as an inflammatory disorder is a relatively recent one. Prior to the 1980s, asthma was considered to result primarily from contraction of the smooth muscles in the airway, and asthma treatment consisted primarily of bronchodilators (medications that expand the bronchi). Medical researchers have made great strides in understanding this disease. Although asthma continues to increase in prevalence throughout many societies, scientists have been moving ahead with new understanding and treatment. It is hoped that these advances will eventually catch up with the galloping rise of the disease and we will see significant decreases in its incidence and severity.

Inflammation is now known to be a key element in the development of asthma, suggesting numerous potential mechanisms by which asthma may be controlled. For example, knowledge of the importance of leukotrienes (you remember them, don't you?) has led to the recent development of antileukotriene agents, the first new class of drugs for the treatment of asthma in twenty-five years. The hope is that new therapies that deal with inflammation by targeting specific molecules involved in asthma will help patients and health-care providers better manage this disease.

# Asthma as an Inflammatory Disease: A Deeper Look

In susceptible individuals, inflammation causes recurrent episodes of wheezing, breathlessness, chest tightness, and cough—particularly at night and/or in the early morning. These symptoms are usually associated with widespread but variable airflow limitation that is at least partly reversible, either spontaneously or with treatment. The inflammation also causes an associated increase in airway responsiveness to a variety of stimuli.

Asthma inflammation is mediated through several different types of inflammatory cells. Among the most major offenders are those produced by the two pathways—cyclo-oxygenase (COX), and lipoxygenase (LOX). The suffix "-ase" at the end of both words means that the offending agents are *enzymes*. Enzymes are proteins that help break down other substances to form new substances. In the case of asthma, there is a series of "breakdown" cells resulting from both pathways. Let's look at a few.

When invaders enter our bodies, our bodies release "fighter" cells to "vanquish" the invaders. Some of these cells are called *eosinophils*. Others are called *monocytes*. These are formed in the bone marrow. They enter the blood and migrate to the connective tissue in the affected area of the body—in this case, the lungs. There, they differentiate into *macrophages*. Picture a macrophage as a sort of cellular "Packman," roving and devouring unwelcome organisms. Additional processes that take place during inflammation are the buildup of blood platelets in contact with the lining of the affected area, the involvement of chemicals released by mast cells, and the shedding of cells along the *epithelium*—the lining.

Let's turn up the lenses on our microscopes by one additional level of magnification and look at the eosinophils. They contain a variety of preformed mediators and, through a series of chemical reactions, they form leukotrienes—the chemicals we've already encountered in the inflammatory process in the joints.

Asthma usually doesn't strike in a vacuum. Typically, it is triggered by an allergic reaction. The food or environmental toxin that triggers this reaction is called an *allergen*. The body releases eosinophils to combat the allergens and these eosinophils, in turn, change to substances that trigger mast cells to release histamine. When you go to the pharmacy to buy an antihistamine to combat some allergic reaction, you're buying a drug that fights histamine. Histamine and leukotrienes have the same impact on the airways leading to the lungs—they cause these airways, which are made of smooth muscle, to contract.

Taking antihistamines might help you stop sneezing if you're allergic to cats and your neighbor just presented you with a kitten. It might help your rash if you have come in contact with poison ivy—which is, ultimately, an allergic reaction to the oils exuded by the poison ivy leaves. By combating histamine, these medications can be crucial and even lifesaving. However, they are not sufficient to combat asthma by themselves. Antihistamines will not address the central role that leukotrienes play in the contraction of the smooth airway muscles—which is an inflammatory response. Leukotrienes are one hundred to one thousand times more bronchoconstricting than histamine! Their effect is also far more prolonged. Leukotrienes don't just lead to the tightening of the bronchial passages. They also stimulate mucus production. They make the tiny blood vessels more permeable, allowing toxins to enter them, and they cause the eosinophils to migrate to new areas, where the inflammatory process starts all over again. This is how they're responsible for the worsening of asthmatic symptoms.

I'll bet that, by now, you can already guess which acid is responsible for leukotriene synthesis. That's right, you've got it! Our old friend, arachidonic acid. And by now you're also a pro in understanding how to reduce the amount of arachidonic acid by adopting dietary and other lifestyle changes. I'm sure you know by now that Lyprinol can play a role in reducing the inflammation associated with asthma . . . but let's not jump too far ahead. Let's continue our study of asthma by looking at existing therapeutic approaches to the disease.

# Current Treatment Approaches to Asthma

Recognition of the important role that inflammation plays in asthma has led to increased emphasis on anti-inflammatory agents to treat the disease. Extensive research efforts are seeking to identify the inflammatory mechanisms associated with asthma and to develop new anti-inflammatory treatments. While control of an asthma attack is still a crucial aspect of asthma therapy, greater attention is being paid to prevention and to management of the chronic inflammatory aspects of the disease.

Asthma is a complex disease in which episodic attacks are superimposed on a chronic inflammatory condition in the lung. The various drugs prescribed by doctors are aimed at different components of the disease. Let's look at a few of the most widely prescribed medications.

## Histamine Receptor Antagonists (Antihistamines)

Histamine is one of the major mediators released from the mast cell in allergic reactions; therefore, preventing its ability to stimulate target organs has become an obvious goal in drug development. Antihistamines are not sufficient to control all aspects of the disease, however, because they do not address the role that leukotrienes play in the vicious cycle of asthma.

## Relievers and Controllers

These are two major categories of drugs aimed at providing relief from asthma symptoms as quickly as possible. As we have seen, asthma is not only a spasm; it's an inflammation—a thickening of the tissue inside the airways. A spasm can be relieved very quickly. If you have a muscle cramp in your calf, for example, some kneading and stretching can bring relief within a matter of seconds. By contrast, inflammation takes much longer to heal. If something is swollen, it may take hours or even days to go down.

RELIEVERS

As the name implies, relievers are designed to bring symptomatic relief. They "despasm" the muscle, so to speak. Bronchodilators dilate or stretch the contracted bronchial muscles. They do not, however, address the full range of symptoms. For example, they are not designed to break up plugs or mucus, or to heal infection. For those purposes, we have a second category of medication, called the *controllers*. The two major controllers are the corticosteroids and the antileukotrienes.

Corticosteroids have been the drug of choice for treating chronic severe asthma since 1950. Although the anti-inflammatory role of steroids was not recognized and understood when these powerful medications were first being prescribed, it is now known that treating milder asthma with corticosteroids may also help to reduce bronchial inflammation and control the progression of the disease. However, systemic corticosteroids, albeit potent and effective medications, have potentially debilitating side effects. They affect the kidneys and the adrenal glands. Some recent research has linked corticosteroids with thyroid disease, mood swings, yeast infections, and a host of other disturbing conditions. And oral corticosteroids are notorious for causing weight gain.

Inhaled corticosteroids are often used as the primary long-term controller therapy for asthma. Although corticosteroid therapy is believed to work by suppressing airway inflammation, it's still not entirely clear exactly how the mechanics of this process work. One study suggested that perhaps corticosteroids reduce the number of inflammatory eosinophils that migrate to the affected tissues. Another theory suggests that corticosteroids may control the production of inflammatory mediators.

Other long-term control therapies are mast cell stabilizers. These seem to inhibit the release of inflammatory mediators by mast cells.

They include DSCG/cromolyn and nedocromil. These medications—which are called *cromones*—are considered safer than corticosteroids because they have a more favorable side-effect profile. However, they are also less effective when it comes to long-term control. Their anti-inflammatory action is only mild, although they are somewhat more versatile than are corticosteroids because they inhibit early phase responses to allergens, as well as chronic allergic-inflammatory reactions.

## BETA-2 AGONISTS

Adrenaline is a beta-2 agonist. It has been used to relieve asthma symptoms for about ninety years. It is a very powerful bronchodilator. It works by selectively activating the beta-2 adrenergic receptors. These are the receptors in the airways that welcome and host adrenaline. When they're activated, they are primed and ready to receive the adrenaline, which can then start to work its magic within the lungs. In fact, short-acting beta-2 agonists are the most powerful bronchodilators available. They include albuterol (Ventolin®, Proventil®), terbutaline, pirbuterol, bitolterol, and levalbuterol. Bronchodilators are delivered by inhalation to ensure rapid onset of action and minimize adverse effects. They are the therapy of choice for relieving acute symptoms and preventing exercise-induced bronchospasm.

Adrenaline also inhibits mast cell mediator secretion and constricts the peripheral blood vessels, causing the heart to pump faster. (In fact, it is the chemical responsible for the "rush" involved in the fight-or-flight response.) However, these are not always desirable effects. Adrenaline (also called epinephrine) places a great strain on the cardiovascular system. People who take the medication report feeling jittery and tense, and many experience palpitations. The consensus at present is that most beta-2 agonists are acceptable as occasional "rescue" remedies but are not suitable for long-term use.

### THEOPHYLLINE

Methylxanthines (extracts from tea and coffee) have been used for almost seven hundred years to treat bronchial asthma. Today the predominant methylxanthine in clinical use is theophylline. Its precise mechanism as an antiasthma drug is somewhat obscure. The biochemical theories behind the drug's effectiveness take us beyond the purview of this book. Suffice it to say here that the major disadvantage with theophylline is that it only works in large doses; but too much theophylline could be toxic. Theophylline also has many undesirable side effects such as excessively rapid heartbeat, high blood pressure, vomiting, seizures, and even death.

# Nonsteroidal Anti-Inflammatory Drugs (NSAIDs)

The use of cyclo-oxygenase (COX) inhibitors such as indomethacin or flurbiprofen inhibits the production of an important *bronchoconstrictor* called $PGD_2$, which is made in the mast cells. While these medications have some beneficial effects during an acute asthma attack induced by allergens, they appear to have little benefit in other forms of chronic asthma. Furthermore, these drugs may precipitate so-called aspirin-induced asthma in a small percentage of patients.

We see that most of the currently available medications contain several major problems. Relievers don't address the root cause of the problem. Controllers bring only limited relief, and many are associated with side effects that can range from moderate to severe.

I'd like to look at the most promising of all currently available asthma medications—the antileukotrienes. I am paying special attention to this class of medication because it appears to have the most long-term effectiveness with the fewest negative effects, and because it is closest in purpose and concept to Lyprinol. After discussing what the antileukotrienes do, we'll look at how they compare to Lyprinol both in terms of effectiveness and in terms of side effects.

# Antileukotrienes

With the realization that inflammation is a key piece in the asthma puzzle, extensive research efforts have gone into identifying the associated inflammatory mechanisms and developing new anti-inflammatory treatments. Through studies of the mechanism of leukotrienes the first new class of drugs for the treatment of asthma in twenty-five years—the antileukotrienes—was developed.

Antileukotriene agents have made asthma compliance much easier. Patients can take them by mouth, rather than by inhaler or injection. They are relatively free of side effects. They're nice, no-fuss-no-muss medications, and they're highly effective to boot.

Antileukotriene agents fall into two general categories: leukotriene synthesis inhibitors (LTSIs) and leukotriene receptor antagonists (LTRAs). LTSIs act at various locations on the leukotriene synthetic pathway; while LTRAs antagonize leukotriene binding at the leukotriene receptors, which are located in the tissues. In other words, LTSIs prevent leukotrienes from being formed in the first place; and if leukotrienes are present, LTRAs prevent them from attaching themselves to the tissues and continuing the inflammatory process.

Although leukotrienes are partially responsible for causing the smooth muscles of the bronchi to contract, for the formation of mucus, and for the increased permeability of the blood vessels, their primary role is in causing inflammation. Studies have shown antileukotrienes to be effective in reducing the number of leukotrienes and inhibiting the effects of those present, even in the presence of allergens that play a role in stimulating leukotriene production.

# Lyprinol versus Antileukotrienes: Which One Wins Out?

Remember our discussion in previous chapters of the science of Lyprinol? Lyprinol acts on the LOX and COX pathways to inhibit all sorts of inflammatory culprits, including leukotrienes. So it stands to reason that Lyprinol should be an effective antiasthmatic agent. But does this assumption hold up under scientific scrutiny?

Let's start by reviewing, once again, the research concerning Lyprinol's effectiveness in healing other inflammatory processes. Dr. Ian Shiels and Dr. Whitehouse compared Lyprinol to two major antileukotrienes (zafirlukast and montelukast). They wanted to see which agent was more effective in relieving arthritis symptoms in laboratory rats. They concluded that both antileukotriene drugs were less effective than Lyprinol. To give you an idea of the difference, zafirlukast inhibited rear paw swelling by 33 percent, and montelukast inhibited it by 71 percent. Lyprinol inhibited rear paw swelling by 96 percent! Combining various measures of arthritis, the doctors arrived at an overall score measuring reduction in arthritis symptoms. The score for zafirlukast was 19; montelukast scored 38, and Lyprinol scored 75. These findings are impressive indeed. Lyprinol also was shown to be more effective than other oils—both plant and marine based.

What does all this have to do with asthma? A great deal, because like arthritis, asthma is an inflammatory process. Leukotrienes play a crucial role in asthma as well as in arthritis. Lyprinol does not confine its activity only to the leukotrienes present in joints and responsible for swelling and pain in your knuckles or knees, for example. It also affects the leukotrienes present in your lungs.

A double-blind placebo-controlled study on asthma was conducted in Saint Petersburg, Russia. The subjects were sixty patients with atopic asthma (asthma associated with allergies) who had never used steroids. The patients were taking "rescue" medications—beta-2 antagonists, such as Proventil®. Lyprinol was given to thirty of these patients at a dosage of two capsules twice a day. The other thirty were in a control group and received a placebo. Lyprinol yielded great improvement in the clinical symptoms of those patients who took it. Improvements were experienced during the night as well as the daytime. There was no similar improvement in the placebo-treated group. The investigators also demonstrated that the bronchial inflammation had been reduced in the Lyprinol group. They concluded that beneficial effects of Lyprinol in mildly asthmatic patients were due to Lyprinol's anti-inflammatory effects on airways. The study is currently being extended to moderate and severe asthma patients. A study of children with moderate asthma is being conducted at the Department of Pediatrics of the same hospital.

Here's another striking aspect of the Saint Petersburg study: Patients who took Lyprinol required their beta-2 antagonist inhalers far less than patients who took the placebo did. This is a powerful and important finding, because—as mentioned above—beta-2 antagonists have potentially serious side effects. Not only is Lyprinol free of side effects, but it also reduces the need for other medications that do have side effects.

So we see that asthma responds nicely to Lyprinol. It appears to be more effective than antileukotrienes. It reduces the need for "rescue" medications that have side effects and, best of all; it has no side effects of its own.

Asthma is usually an allergic process. It is an inflammation that arises as a result of the presence of allergens in the body. Is Lyprinol as effective in combating other allergic processes, such as sneezing, or allergic rashes? Let's look at the evidence.

# Lyprinol and Allergies

The mechanisms of allergy are not fully understood, although scientists are beginning to fill in many of the missing pieces of the puzzle. In order to grasp what the current research has to say, it is important to understand what an allergy is, and what happens in the body when an allergen invades.

As mentioned, our bodies have an immune system designed to fight invading organisms. Without this immune system, we would fall prey to every illness floating around. In fact, people who are born with diseases that rob them of immunity must live their lives in protective "bubbles" where all foreign organisms can be filtered out. The Acquired Immune Deficiency Syndrome (AIDS) virus robs its victims of their ability to fight off illness. Patients therefore are vulnerable to all sorts of "opportunistic infections"—invading organisms that take advantage of the body's inability to fight them off. So our immune system is a gift and something to be grateful for.

But when the immune system goes awry and begins attacking "friendly" invaders, we have a phenomenon known as allergies. It would be as if the border patrol of a country began taking shots not only at armed and obviously hostile enemy invaders but also at friendly visitors from other countries who arrive with peaceful intentions, seeking to tour the United States, or to immigrate. So a person allergic to citrus fruits will react to orange juice as if it were, say, an invading cold virus—by sneezing or sniffling, for example. This might be called a sort of biochemical xenophobia turned inward.

How does this process work? Every offending substance releases an *antigen*—a protein or carbohydrate substance capable of stimulating an immune response. The body responds by releasing *antibodies*—these are proteins produced by specialized "B" cells after they have been prodded by the presence of the antigen. The antibodies are designed to fight the antigens. The main class of antibody associated with allergy is *Immunoglobulin E (IgE)*. Interestingly, that is also the class of antibody responsible for fighting parasites. If you have a case of ringworm, for example, your body will put out a lot of IgE. Is this just coincidence that the same group of antibodies responsible for combating parasites is also responsible for combating allergens? Scientists don't think so. It appears that there actually are tiny living organisms in some apparently inanimate allergens. These microscopic organisms trigger the body's release of those antibodies that fight parasites. For example, dust—a very common allergen—would appear to be inanimate. What could be alive in a pile of dust? In reality, however, thousands of tiny dust *mites* live in the dust. Allergic individuals are not reacting to the dust itself but to the mites in the dust.

IgE production is regulated by a series of messengers that we call cytokines (*cyto* is a cell, and *kine* means move). These cytokines carry the message from the antigens released by the allergen to the cells that produce IgE. The messenger responsible for boosting the production of IgE in allergic patients is called interleukin-4 (IL-4).

"Kill the messenger" may be an inhumane policy when it comes to war and foreign relations, but it's a highly effective policy when it comes to cytokines. It is desirable to slow or destroy IL-4 so that it can't deliver its message to the cells that produce IgE.

IL-4 is not the only messenger on the stage. The allergy process is complex—it's not a monologue, a one-person show. Picture an allergic reaction as a group of many actors who come and go. A leukotriene called leukotriene $B_4$ ($LTB_4$) is the producer and director of the show. It recruits and organizes the actors and gives them their stage commands. The research of Paris-based scientist Dr. Bernard Dugas showed that Lyprinol slows down the activity of IL-4 *and* that it reduces $LTB_4$. There is therefore a much weaker "recruiter" to marshal the actors, and no messengers available to transmit the recruiter's instructions. Without a recruiter and a messenger, the IgE-producing cells don't proceed with antibody production, and no allergic reaction takes place.

The implications of Dugas's work are far-reaching indeed. They suggest that Lyprinol is effective not only in allergic reactions such as asthma but also in other allergic reactions, such as skin rashes. Let's have a closer look at Lyprinol's effectiveness in helping those who suffer from allergy-induced skin disorders.

## *Dermatitis*

Dermatitis is an inflammation of the skin. It can take many different forms, including swelling, redness, itching, burning, and rashes of different shapes, textures, and sizes. Lyprinol has been shown to be effective in relieving both atopic and contact dermatitis. Let's look at each in turn.

## ATOPIC DERMATITIS (INFANTILE ECZEMA)

Atopic dermatitis (AD) is a chronic, itchy rash that progresses into open, oozing sores. It is caused by an overactive immune system. About 2 percent of the total population may have atopic dermatitis. It is a disease that favors youth—the majority of patients are infants and children.

The clinical characteristics of atopic dermatitis are:

- It affects >2 percent of total population—80 to 90 percent affected are 5 years of age.
- It's associated with asthma and allergic rhinitis.
- There is hyperirritability of the skin (pruritus).
- Scratching makes it worse and also maintains inflammation.

The clinical manifestations of the disease—both the type of skin lesions as well as their distribution—typically change with age. They can range from acute to mild, and they can be transient or chronic. AD is not a steady-state disease; patients will cycle from periods of extreme involvement to times when they are symptom-free. This makes treating the disease frustrating.

The skin of patients with atopic dermatitis is in a constant state of hyperirritability, and itching is the main manifestation that bothers patients. Patients can't seem to stop scratching. The scratching worsens the condition, and a vicious cycle ensues. I call it the chronic itch-scratch cycle. It maintains and worsens the inflammation. While atopic dermatitis affects people of all ages, babies and young children are especially vulnerable, because it is hardest to stop them from scratching. You cannot reason with them verbally, and it is difficult to physically restrain them.

Unlike other allergic reactions, which involve IgE-mediated mechanisms, atopic dermatitis appears to involve other antibodies. There are other inflammatory substances that infiltrate the skin.

These include *lympho-histiocytic* cells. Tiny *vesicles* form in the outer layer of the skin, the epidermis. There is no obvious involvement of mast cells, nor is there an obvious presence of eosinophils.

Does this mean that there is no IgE or eosinophil involvement in atopic dermatitis whatsoever? Research suggests that there may be some initial role played by eosinophils. Patients with severe generalized atopic dermatitis tend to have very high total serum IgE concentrations. This means that although no IgE is found at the location of the rash, there is a great deal of IgE circulating in their blood systems that is easily identifiable in blood tests. Individuals who suffer from atopic dermatitis tend to produce high concentrations of IgE when they are exposed to common inhalants and even to certain foods. Sufferers from AD have noticed that when they come in close contact with animals to which they are allergic, they develop a runny nose or asthma. Some develop eczema around the eyes and nose during pollen season. We know that these types of allergic reactions *are* mediated by the mast cells, through the inflammatory processes we discussed in connection with asthma. So, although some AD patients have normal IgE concentrations, the overlap between those who suffer from AD and those who suffer from other IgE-mediated allergies is too large to be coincidental. It seems likely that the release of leukotrienes during other allergic reactions worsens the AD.

Lyprinol can be helpful in combating AD, as we will see below.

## CONTACT DERMATITIS

Allergic contact dermatitis (ACD), a form of delayed hypersensitivity, is a common dermatological problem. If we apply an allergen to the skin of a sensitive patient, an eczematous reaction, localized to the area of the hypersensitivity response, will develop within one to three days.

Common contact allergens include:

- metals such as nickel and cobalt in earring studs, buckles, zippers, fasteners, or jean studs
- latex
- animal hair and dander
- chromium salts in cement, tanned leather, green textile dyes
- para-phenylenediamine (a black dye extracted from coal that is often found in hair dye and some clothing)
- medicinal ointments, such as neomycin and synthetic local anesthetics
- epoxy resins, fragrances in soaps and toiletries, and creams and ointments containing wood alcohols and parabens

In many parts of the world, nickel is the most common offending allergen, especially in women with pierced ears. Ingested nickel (occasionally found in water or in poorly maintained cookware) may cause dermatitis in skin that has previously been in contact with nickel.

Common allergens differ from continent to continent. In North America, for example, poison oak and poison ivy are common causes of ACD.

Causes of ACD may be immediately apparent or may take considerable sleuthing to define, especially when caused by industrial processes.

## Lyprinol and Dermatitis

There has been a good deal of research focusing on Lyprinol's impact on dermatitis. But before we review the studies, a brief introduction regarding skin research is in order.

How do cosmetic manufacturers determine whether a new product is safe for the skin? They perform a test called the Kligman-

Magnusson, which is standard for the cosmetic and dermatological industries. Shaved guinea pigs are exposed to a substance to see if they become allergic to it. If they develop a negative skin reaction—contact dermatitis—it is assumed that human beings may also develop contact dermatitis from that substance.

Once shaved guinea pigs are suffering from contact dermatitis induced by exposure to an allergen, scientists apply various substances to determine whether they are effective in relieving the symptoms of the allergic reaction. As you will see, Dr. Michael Whitehouse followed these protocols in ascertaining the effectiveness of Lyprinol in relieving contact dermatitis.

Dr. Whitehouse made two fascinating discoveries regarding the role Lyprinol can play in relieving symptoms of both types of dermatitis. He demonstrated that a topical preparation of Lyprinol cured existing dermatitis in animals such as shaved guinea pigs almost as fast as corticosteroids did. Even more impressive, he discovered that if he gave Lyprinol to these animals orally, they did not develop dermatitis when exposed to allergens. Dr. Whitehouse's topical preparation requires some fine-tuning if it is to be used effectively for human beings, because it has a foul odor. Research on a more pleasantly aromatic topical formulation is under way. Meanwhile, you can use oral Lyprinol to offset your allergic responses to skin irritants.

We have seen that Lyprinol is effective in relieving both asthma and dermatitis. How about other manifestations of allergy, such as sneezing, runny nose, itchy and watery eyes, and congestion? Let's examine the evidence.

### Allergic Rhinitis (AR)

Rhinitis is not a disease that afflicts the rhinoceros. It is the medical term for those nasty respiratory symptoms you associate with colds—runny nose, nasal congestion, itching, and sneezing. And have you ever wondered whether it's a cold or an allergy? Whether it's some type of upper-respiratory infection, the pollen outside, or the neighbor's cat? Here are a few questions to help you decide:

- Is there a family history of allergies?

- What is your dominant nasal symptom? Is it blockage, sneezes, or runny nose?

- Are the nasal problems isolated, or are there more extensive symptoms? For example, what is happening in other parts of the upper airways, such as sinuses or ears? Have you ever suffered from bronchitis, ear infections, or skin problems? A history of bronchitis and ear infections, for example, might suggest that a persistent cough or an itchy ear is due to an infection. If you have a rash together with your itchy ears, an allergy seems more likely—especially if you're not prone to ear infections.

- Look around your house. Is it cluttered with lots of "soft" items, such as blankets, carpets, and stuffed toys? Do you have pets? Do you keep flowering plants in the house? How about outdoors? What types of vegetation grow in your neighborhood? Are you near some type of industrial plant, or other source of air pollution?

- What are your occupation and leisure activities, and do they aggravate your symptoms?

- Can you find any connection between your symptoms and what you eat or drink?

These questions are designed to give you clues as to what may be going on. Of course, this is not an exhaustive list. If you have any doubt, you should consult your health-care practitioner. If infection is ruled out and your AR symptoms don't disappear, you might consult an allergist or an expert in environmental medicine. These specialists are skilled in ferreting out clues you may not have thought of, and testing for reactions to specific substances.

Allergic sensitization seems to occur in very early life when the immune system is immature. Maybe this is the reason why allergic rhinitis is more common in those born in the spring and summer. There is also a higher prevalence of rhinitis in boys than in girls— possibly a genetically determined difference, since IgE levels are higher in boys from birth. Firstborn children are at greatest risk. The relative risk is doubled for children who live in damp houses and/or whose parents smoke. Modern energy-efficient "tight" buildings increase exposure to potential allergens. Environmental pollution is likewise a prime offender.

Recent studies have shown that the antileukotrienes are effective against AR—especially when used in conjunction with antihistamines. People who have tried using Lyprinol together with their antihistamine report that they get far more relief than they did from self-standing antihistamines. While formal scientific studies have not yet been conducted regarding the effectiveness of Lyprinol in alleviating symptoms of AR, the testimonials of those who have tried it are impressive.

"My Kleenex bill is way down," said one satisfied Lyprinol user. "I can finally smell the roses!" said another. A third spoke enthusiastically of increased energy and relief from exercise-induced asthma. "I plan to run the New York Marathon!" he announced.

One patient reported relief from nighttime congestion and resultant snoring. "Maybe I should look for a wife," he quipped.

# Speaking of Allergies . . . Has Anyone Ever Been Allergic to Lyprinol?

Lyprinol is nonallergenic!

To start with, there is no protein and no carbohydrate present in Lyprinol. Since these are the types of foods that classically induce allergies, the risk of allergy to Lyprinol is nonexistent.

I have sometimes been contacted by patients who are concerned that they may react poorly to Lyprinol because they are allergic to mussels. I investigated this by contacting the director of the European Research Center on Food Allergies in Nancy, France. My researches have led me to believe that this is the finest and most sophisticated center for the study of food allergies in the world. Professor Anne-Denise Moneret-Vautrin, the director of the center, told me that even people who are allergic to mussels will not develop an allergy to mussel oil. She assured me that there is no evidence of IgE-related reactions to any type of mussel oil. Moreover, she has never encountered even a single documented case of such a reaction. The absence of protein and carbohydrate in the oil means that there is no chemical "welcoming committee" for an IgE reaction. So Lyprinol is safe for you, even if you don't tolerate shellfish.

# 7

•

# Lyprinol and Women's Health

Women are different from men. I'm not talking about subtle difference in communicational styles or planetary origins (Mars versus Venus). Women are biochemically different from men. They have unique needs emanating from their hormonal cycles. In particular, many women suffer from pain and discomfort during their menstrual period. Lyprinol has been proven highly effective in addressing *dysmenorrhea*—painful menstrual periods. Up to 50 percent of menstruating women suffer primary dysmenorrhea at significant economic and social cost. In the United States it has been estimated that 600 million work hours are lost each year due to dysmenorrhea. Heather is an example of a woman whose quality of life was seriously compromised by dysmenorrhea, and who used Lyprinol successfully to address her symptoms.

- *Heather is a thirty-eight-year-old laboratory technician. Like all the women in her family, she suffered from "bad veins." She had varicose veins in her legs and uncomfortable hemorrhoids.*

*Due to her vascular problems, her high cholesterol, and a predi-abetic condition, she could not use oral contraceptives, so her gynecologist inserted an intrauterine device (IUD) in her uterus for birth control.*

*Heather began experiencing terrible pelvic pain beginning three to four days prior to her period, which worsened during menstruation. She had to take off from work ten days each month. Ibuprofen led to a life-threatening uterine hemorrhage, and did nothing to alleviate the pain. Other medications she tried caused a host of nasty side effects, including nausea, constipation, mood swings, and dizziness.*

*Heather started taking four capsules of Lyprinol daily ten days before her period was expected and discontinued on the last day of her period. For the first time, she experienced no pain, cramps, or excessive bleeding. She followed the same protocol the following month and has continued doing so ever since. She no longer misses work during her menstrual period and reports feeling enormous relief.*

How does Lyprinol alleviate the pain and discomfort associated with menstruation? First let's understand what dysmenorrhea is—and what it isn't.

When we are in pain, we tend to think that something is wrong. We associate physical discomfort with illness. But actually, dysmenorrhea is usually not caused by an illness. Rather, it is associated with increased levels of prostaglandins and/or lipoxygenase (LOX-produced) leukotrienes—both of which are inflammatory substances, but both of which are also the mediators of uterine contractions.

As part of its normal physiological function, the uterus contracts rhythmically during menstruation. The force and frequency of these contractions are regulated by the sex hormones—specifically, oxytocin, a hormone synthesized in the pituitary gland. (That's the same hormone that doctors and midwives use to intensify the contractions of women whose labor is progressing too slowly.) Oxytocin stimulates strong uterine contractions, and it also acts to increase the local release of eicosanoids.

Elevated concentrations of all classes of eicosanoids such as prostaglandins and leukotrienes have been identified in women suffering from dysmenorrhea. These mediators increase the force of uterine contractions (more commonly called cramps) and constrict blood vessels. They make pain receptors in the pelvic area exquisitely sensitive to all kinds of physical stimuli or chemicals that induce pain. Under ordinary circumstances, these receptors would be more likely to ignore those stimuli. Now, they're all on red alert.

But that's not all they do . . .

The eicosanoids enter the circulation and cause general malaise often accompanied by diarrhea, headache, dizziness, and nausea.

Why does the body release these hormones during menstruation? Prostaglandins and leukotrienes are physiological mediators of normal uterine contractions and are necessary during menstruation so that the blood will be expelled by the uterus. But when too much production of prostaglandins and leukotrienes takes place, the uterine contractions become too strong and pain develops. While this experience can range from mild discomfort to "please-let-me-lie-down" agony, it is not in and of itself dangerous or pathological.

On the other hand, it's not desirable either. Pain is useful only when it signals the presence of an illness or condition that needs attention. For example, if you break your ankle and experience no pain, you might put weight on the broken bone and worsen the break, rendering your ankle permanently useless. If you come down with strep throat but feel no throat pain, you might never know you have the illness and might end up suffering all the potentially dangerous conditions associated with untreated strep. However here, there's no illness being signaled, and therefore no good reason to suffer.

What will relieve the pain?

Approximately 80 percent of women with dysmenorrhea experience symptomatic relief when they are treated with one of the NSAIDs that inhibit the COX enzymes responsible for synthesizing prostaglandins. However, NSAIDs do not give satisfactory relief in approximately 20 percent of primary dysmenorrhea patients. (Heather is an example of a patient who could not take NSAIDs.) And of course, NSAIDs have negative side effects, as we discussed earlier. It is common practice to use oral contraceptives to treat these women—but even oral contraceptives are not free of risks.

With the help of Lyprinol, it may be possible to reduce the pain you feel during your periods, even without NSAIDs and oral contraceptives. Drs. Ian Shiels and Michael Whitehouse studied uterine contractions in rats. They showed that administering Lyprinol to uterine tissue reduces uterine contractions—even when those contractions have been artificially induced by administration of oxytocin.

Why does Lyprinol have this effect on uterine contractions? Studies show that Lyprinol is not a smooth-muscle relaxant, nor does it inhibit any of the chemicals produced by the COX pathway. Rather, it seems to work against the leukotriene receptors in the uterus. If these receptors are blocked, the leukotriene can't exert its contractive effect on the uterus, and the uterus will consequently be more relaxed.

There is some anecdotal evidence to support the use of Lyprinol for dysmenorrhea in human beings. Several women suffering from arthritis were taking Lyprinol to alleviate the inflammation in their joints. Some of them also suffered from dysmenorrhea, but did not realize that Lyprinol might alleviate their menstrual discomforts. They were surprised to discover dramatic reductions in their symptoms of dysmenorrhea after they started taking Lyprinol.

Lyprinol is safe for women who are taking oral contraceptives. There is no risk of either excessive clotting or of excessive bleeding, even for women who are wearing intrauterine devices (IUDs).

# 8

●

# New Directions of Lyprinol Research: What's on the Horizon?

We have talked about Lyprinol as a powerful and effective remedy for arthritis, cardiovascular disease, asthma, and allergies. There are a variety of other situations and conditions in which Lyprinol can be helpful. Scientists studying Lyprinol are expanding their investigations into all sorts of new areas. Here are a few of the far-reaching possibilities currently under investigation:

# Working with Vaccines to Strengthen Immunity

A fascinating double-blind, placebo-controlled study was conducted in 1999—a collaborative project between Russian and Australian scientists concerning the impact that four weeks of Lyprinol supplementation might have on the response to influenza vaccination. Subjects were vaccinated with a live, weakened nasal vaccine. The findings implied that Lyprinol might independently decrease the unwanted inflammatory reaction that we develop when we suffer from the flu (that "achiness" in our joints, for example). Taken together with the vaccine, Lyprinol greatly strengthened the effectiveness of the vaccine. And Lyprinol didn't have any negative impact on the normal immune response.

# Lyprinol: The Next Cure for Cancer?

In 1998 and 1999, Dr. Betts from Australia applied Lyprinol to several lines of cancer cells. He was excited to discover that those cells died within twenty-four hours. They underwent apoptosis, or programmed cell death. What followed was a great media hubbub, with Lyprinol touted as the upcoming cure for cancer. While there is great hope that Lyprinol might indeed provide a natural alternative for cancer treatment without the side effects of chemotherapy and radiation, that day has not yet arrived. Research is under way, and anecdotal reports have been encouraging. Patients have reported that tumors have shrunk or at least remained unchanged, and that tumor markers have stabilized or decreased. Many patients have experienced relief from pain and a return of appetite. All in all, they report that their quality of life has improved. It remains to be seen whether the enthusiastic reports of satisfied patients will be confirmed by thorough scientific studies.

# Inflammatory Bowel Disease

As the name implies, inflammatory bowel disease (IBD) is an inflammatory disorder of the digestive tract. It stands to reason that anti-inflammatory agents will alleviate the symptoms of this condition—and that's the rationale behind supplementation with omega-3 PUFAs, which (as you know by now) have anti-inflammatory effects in the body. In fact, the first evidence of the importance of dietary intake of omega-3 polyunsaturated fatty acids was derived from epidemiological observations of the low incidence of inflammatory bowel disease in Eskimos.

Crohn's disease is an example of an inflammatory bowel disorder that may be responsive to Lyprinol. The disease is a chronic inflammation of the intestinal tract. Two gastroenterologists in Australia gave Lyprinol to two of their patients who suffered from Crohn's disease—with highly encouraging results. The patients now have normal barium X rays, and physical examination of the rectal area shows no sign of disease. These physicians were so impressed by these promising results that they are planning to conduct a more formal and extensive study.

# Diabetes

Diabetes is not a single disease entity. Rather, it's a group of diseases characterized by the body's inability to produce sufficient quantities of insulin. The pancreas doesn't make enough insulin, or doesn't make any insulin at all. Sometimes, the pancreas produces enough insulin but the body is unable to utilize that insulin properly.

Insulin is the most important hormone involved in metabolism of your food. It helps use glucose from carbohydrates. Cells use this glucose to produce energy to grow and function. Diabetics are unable to use the sugars they eat because they lack the ability to metabolize them.

Diabetes has been associated with high levels of one particular category of blood fat—the triglycerides. Studies conducted over a ten-year period show that fish-oil supplementation for patients with type II diabetes lowers triglycerides *without* adversely affecting blood-sugar levels. These data suggest that a marine oil such as Lyprinol may be safe to add to triglyceride-lowering medication for people with diabetes.

# Multiple Sclerosis (MS)

Lyprinol might be helpful in treating MS—an autoimmune disease that affects the central nervous system (brain and spinal cord). MS occurs when inflammation destroys the insulating myelin sheath that covers the nerve fibers. The nerves lose much of their protective coating. It would be as if the thick plastic coating on phone or electrical wires is stripped away, leaving exposed areas. In the brain, these areas of scarring are called scleroses. The damage in these scleroses slows or blocks muscle coordination, visual sensation, and other nerve signals.

Dr. Sheila Gibson, at the Western Glasgow Hospital in Scotland, is currently studying whether Lyprinol has a beneficial impact on patients with MS who did not respond to any previous treatments. While the effectiveness of Lyprinol in combating inflammatory symptoms of MS appears to be logical, only empirical and scientifically valid evidence will prove whether that contention is correct.

I hope that this chapter has whetted your interest in following news reports emanating from the scientific community regarding the many fascinating applications of Lyprinol. I believe we are living in exciting times and that the studies currently under way are at the cutting edge of modern research into nonpharmaceutical management of chronic illness.

# 9

•

# How to Use Lyprinol: A Guide for the Consumer

We have seen how Lyprinol works and what it can do. Now it's time for some practical advice regarding its use.

## Recommended Dosages

Whether you're suffering from arthritis, asthma, or circulatory problems, the recommended course of Lyprinol treatment is:

- Four capsules a day at first
- After one month, or after you experience symptom relief, cut dosage in half.

- After another month, cut dosage in half again.
- This is your maintenance dosage (one capsule a day).

Many of the variables that affect the response seem to include the amount of omega-6 oils you have consumed in the past, and that you continue to consume; and the amount of other inflammatory processes at work in your body (allergies, asthma, heart and circulatory problems, diabetes, etc).

It takes a month or more for the omega-3 fatty acids to build up in the body. Patients must therefore take the largest quantity of Lyprinol at the beginning of treatment, and then gradually decrease the dosage until they reach a level that will maintain the desired effects.

# Further Tips for Lyprinol Use

Here are some additional guidelines:

- Take Lyprinol during meals. Some people have reported experiencing mild nausea when they took Lyprinol on an empty stomach.
- Take two capsules during breakfast and two during dinner.
- Even if you are suffering from acute inflammation, don't increase the dose.
- The dose should remain the same even if you're already taking some other medication, such as an NSAID.

# How Can You Obtain Lyprinol?

Lyprinol is available in the United States and Canada by mail or phone order. It may be obtained through:

**Tyler Encapsulations, Inc.**
9725 SW Commerce Circle, Suite A-9
Wilsonville, OR 97070
Phone: (800) 869-9705
www.tyler-inc.com
e-mail: hankc@tyler-inc.com or info@tyler-inc.com

Lyprinol is available at a number of health food stores under its retail brand name Prevail. Details regarding locations of such stores can be provided by calling 1-800-248-0885, or you can order Prevail Lyprinol by calling 1-800-681-7099, where credit card orders are accepted. The product is distributed by:

**Enzymatic Therapy**
825 Challenger Drive
Green Bay, WI 54311
Phone: (800) 783-2286
www.enzy.com
e-mail: etmail@enzy.com

Lyprinol is also distributed through health-care providers, so you may want to check with yours.

Finally, Lyprinol is also distributed by Life Plus International, a network marketing company that sells through distributors who sell under the name Lyprinex™. Life Plus has offices in the U.S. and Europe.

**Life Plus International**
P.O. Box 3749
Batesville, AR 72501
Phone: (800) 572-8446
www.lifeplus.com

**Life Plus Europe**
Life Plus House, Little End Road
Eaton Socon, Cambridgeshire
PE19 8JH England
Phone: 44 1480 477 230

You can also contact:

**Pharmalink Marketing Services Pty. Ltd.**
19 Taree Street
Burleigh Heads, Queensland 42220
Australia
Phone: 011-61-7-5568-8250
Fax: 011-61-7-5522-0822
e-mail: pharma@onthenet.com.au

# Can Lyprinol Go Stale?

The shelf life of most gelatin capsules is usually five years. Theoretically, they are totally weatherproof and impermeable to air. As of July 2000, the oldest batches of Lyprinol were two years old, and there was no degradation and no modification in the capsule. So we know that after two years the oils are still active, they have not been oxidized, and there are no changes. To play it safe twice, although Lyprinol is an antioxidant as defined by the pharmaceutical industry, the industry always adds less than a quarter of a milligram of additional antioxidant (alpha-tocopherol, which is vitamin E) to these gelatin soft capsules. This trace of vitamin E is enough to prevent oxidation. But be warned: The amount of vitamin E in a capsule of Lyprinol is minuscule, so don't substitute this vitamin E for your regular vitamin supplement! The amount is far too small to have any effect on you.

Store Lyprinol in a cool, dry place so that it doesn't get gummy.

# 10

•

# Conclusions

If you have taken this book off your library or bookstore shelf, you have shown that you are interested in improving your health, or helping someone in your family who suffers from a chronic inflammatory illness. I hope this information will indeed be helpful to you, or will enable you to assist your loved one.

Even if you are not currently suffering from one of the illnesses discussed in this book, I hope that you will consider using Lyprinol preventively. It can only enhance your health. In fact, there really is no "down" side to taking Lyprinol. All the studies have demonstrated that you cannot overdose on Lyprinol, nor will it interact negatively with herbs, other supplements, or medications.

Of course, as mentioned earlier, Lyprinol is not a magic bullet. It will work best when it is incorporated into a broader health-improvement plan, including a well-balanced diet, regular exercise, and a low-stress lifestyle. I believe that these recommendations comprise the formula for good health.

In the words of the Maori, "Kia pai o koutou oranga!"—or "Be in good health."

# Appendix A:
# Composition of
# Lyprinol Capsules

| Materials | mg/capsule |
|---|---|
| **Fill Materials:** | |
| Lyprinol extract | 50.000 |
| Olive oil, food grade | 100.775 |
| D Alpha Tocopherol 1,000 iu/qusp | 0.225 |
| | |
| **Shell Materials** | |
| Glycerine BP | 16.340 |
| Sorbitol Syrup 70% BP | 22.120 |
| Gelatin 150 bloom BP | 58.340 |
| | |
| *Content of Heavy Metals* | *mg/capsule* |
| Cadmium | <0.01 |
| Mercury | <0.01 |

| | |
|---|---|
| Lead | <0.05 |
| Arsenic | <0.50 |
| Copper | 0.16 |
| Tin | <0.10 |
| Zinc | <0.41 |
| Iron | 2.20 |
| Selenium | <0.10 |

Method of determination—atomic absorption spectrometry using flame and hybrid generation.

| Residue of Pesticides (mg/kg) | mg/capsule |
|---|---|
| Organochlorine pesticides | <0.02 |
| Organophosphorus type pesticides | <0.02 |

Method of determination—capillary GC with ECD and ND method sensivity—0.02 ppm.

*Microbiological Burden*

| TEST TYPE | RESULT | TEST UNIT | FHL LQM NO. |
|---|---|---|---|
| Total plate count | <10 | CFU/g | Method MFH001 |
| Coliform count | Nil | MPN/g | Method MFH005 |
| *Clostridium perfringens* | <100 | CFU/g | Method MFH013 |
| *Bacillus cereus* | <100 | CFU/g | Method MFH010 |
| *Salmonella* spp. | Not detected in 25g | | |
| Anaerobic count | <10 | CFU/g | |

*Additives*
None

# Appendix A: Composition of Lyprinol Capsules

*Nutritional analysis*

| | |
|---|---|
| Energy | 6 kj/capsule |
| | 1.3 cal/capsule |
| Protein | 0 mg/capsule |
| Fat | 150 mg/capsule |
| Saturated fatty acids | 30 mg/capsule |
| Unsaturated fatty acids | 30 mg/capsule |
| Eicosatetraenoic acid (ETA) | 0.17 mg/capsule |
| Carbohydrate | 0 mg/capsule |

## Vitamins        150 ng/capsule

## Cholesterol        195 µg/capsule

(Note: This amount is quite small when compared to items such as 213 mg of cholesterol in one egg.)

# Appendix B: Nonsteroidal Anti-Inflammatory Drugs (NSAIDs)

The conventional medical treatments for arthritis have largely involved analgesics and nonsteroidal anti-inflammatory drugs (NSAIDs). These are designed to control the symptoms of arthritis, including pain and stiffness. Some of these compounds are prescription drugs while others are over-the-counter remedies. The principal and significant drawback of these drugs is their tendency to ulcerate the mucous membranes of the stomach and intestinal tract. Some 25 percent of patients experience one or more of numerous serious side effects, which range from bleeding ulcers, stomach and intestinal discomfort, to liver and kidney problems, and even death.

NSAIDs available on the market (both prescription and nonprescription) include:

Aches-N-pain
Advil
Advil Caplets

Albert-Tiafen
Alka Butazolidin
Alkabutazone

Alka-Phenylbutazone
Alrheumat
Amersol
Anaprox
Anaprox-Ds
Ansaid
Apo-Diclo
Apo-Flurbiprofen
Apo-Ibuprofen
Apo-Indomethacin
Apo-Keto
Apo-Keto-E
Apo-Naproxen
Apo-Piroxicam
Apsifen
Apsifen-F
Bayer Select Pain Relief
   Formula Caplets
Brufen
Butacote
Butazone
Children's Advil
Clinoril
CoAdvil
Cotybutazone
Cramp End
Diclofenac
Diflunisal
Dolgesic
Dolobid
Etodolac
Excedrin-IB

Feldene
Fenoprofen
Fenopron
Flurbiprofen
Froben
Genpril
Haltran
Ibifon 600
Ibren
Ibu
Ibu-4
Ibu-6
Ibu-8
Ibu-200
Ibumed
Ibuprin
Ibupro-600
Ibuprofen
Ibutex
Ifen
Imbrilon
Indameth
Indocid
Indocid SR
Indocin
Indocin SR
Indolar SR
Indomethacin
Intrabutazone
Ketoprofen
Lidifen
Lodine

Meclofen
Meclofenamate
Meclomen
Medipren
Mefenamic Acid
Midol 200
Midol IB
Motrin
Motrin IB
Motrin IB caplets
Motrin, Children's
Nabumetone
Nalfon
Nalfon 200
Naprosyn
Naproxen
Naxen
Novobutazone
Novo-Keto-EC
Novomethacin
Novonaprox
Novopirocam
Novoprofen
Novo-Sundac
Nu-Indo
Nu-Pirox
Nuprin
Orudis
Orudis-E

Oruvail
Pamprin-IB
Paxofen
Pedia
Phenylbutazone
Phenylone Plus
Piroxicam
Ponstan
Ponstel
Progesic
Relafen
Rhodis-EC
Rufen
Saleto-200
Saleto-400
Saleto-600
Saleto-800
Sulindac
Surgam
Synflex
Telectin DS
Tenoxicam
Tiaprofenic acid
Tolmetin
Trendar
Voltaren
Voltaren SR
Voltarol
Voltarol Retard

# Selected References

Adler, A. J., and B. J. Holub. "Effect of Garlic and Fish-Oil Supplementation on Serum Lipid and Lipoprotein Concentrations in Hypercholesterolemic Men," *American Journal of Clinical Nutrition* 64 (1997): 445–450.

Antileukotriene Working Group, Leff, A. D. et al. *Asthma 2000— The Role of Antileukotrienes in Clinical Practice.* October 1999, Discovery International.

Audeval, B., and P. Bouchacourt. "Etude contrôlée, en double aveugle contre placebo, de l'extrait de moule *Perna canaliculus* (moule aux orles verts) dans la gonarthrose." *La Gazette Médicale* 93 (1986):111–16.

Bang, H. O., and J. Dyerberg. "Plasma Lipids and Lipoproteins in Greenlandic West Coast Eskimos." *Acta Medica Scandinavica* 192(1972):85–94.

Belluzzi, A., S. Boschi, C. Brignola, A. Munarini, G. Cariani, and F. Miglio. "Polyunsaturated Fatty Acids and Inflammatory Bowel

Disease." *American Journal of Clinical Nutrition* 71(2000):339S–342S.

Bhathena, S. J., E. Berlin, J. T. Judd, Y. C. Kim, J. S. Law, H. N. Bhagavan, R. Ballard-Barbash, and P. P. Nair. "Effects of Omega-3 Fatty Acids and Vitamin E on Hormones Involved in Carbohydrate and Lipid Metabolism in Men." *American Journal of Clinical Nutrition* 54(1991):684–88.

Blonk, M. C., H. J. Bilo, J. J. Nauta, C. Popp-Snijders, C. Mulder, and A. J. Donker. "Dose-Response Effects of Fish-Oil Supplementation in Healthy Volunteers." *American Journal of Clinical Nutrition* 52(1990):120–27.

Burr, M. L. "Lessons from the Story of Omega-3 Fatty Acids." *American Journal of Clinical Nutrition* 71(2000):397S–398S.

Cobiac, L., P. M. Clifton, M. Abbey, G. B. Belling, and P. J. Nestel. "Lipid, Lipoprotein, and Hemostatic Effects of Fish vs. Fish-Oil Omega-3 Fatty Acids in Mildly Hyperlipidemic Males." *American Journal of Clinical Nutrition* 53(1991):1210–16.

Connor, S. L. and W. E. Connor. "Are Fish Oils Beneficial in the Prevention and Treatment of Coronary Artery Disease?" *American Journal of Clinical Nutrition* 66(1997)1020S–1031S.

Connor, W. E. "Importance of Omega-3 Fatty Acids in Health and Disease." *American Journal of Clinical Nutrition* 71(2000)171S–175S.

Connor, W. E., and A. Bendich, eds. "Highly Unsaturated Fatty Acids in Nutrition and Disease Prevention." Proceedings of conference held in Barcelona, Spain, November 4–6, 1996. Supplement to *American Journal of Clinical Nutrition* 71(2000).

Dannenberg, A. J., and D. Zakim. "Chemoprevention of Colorectal Cancer Through Inhibition of Cyclooxygenase-2." *Seminars in Oncology* 26(1999):499–504.

Donadio, J. V., Jr. "Use of Fish Oil to Treat Patients with Immuno-globulin A. Nephropathy." *American Journal of Clinical Nutrition* 71(2000)373S–375S.

Dugas, B. "Lyprinol Inhibits $LTB_4$ Production by Human Monocytes." *Allergie & Immunologie* 32(2000)284–89.

Fernandez, E., L. Chatenoud, C. La Vecchia, E. Negri, and S. Franceschi. "Fish Consumption and Cancer Risk." *American Journal of Clinical Nutrition* 70(1999):85–90.

Flaten, H., A. T. Hostmark, P. Kierulf, E. Lystad, K. Trygg, T. Bjerkedal, and A. Osland. "Fish-Oil Concentrate: Effects on Variables Related to Cardiovascular Disease." *American Journal of Clinical Nutrition* 52(1990):300–306.

Gibson, R. G., S. L. M. Gibson, V. Conway, and D. Chappell. "*Perna Canaliculus* in the Treatment of Arthritis." *The Practitioner* 224(1980)955–960.

Gibson, S. L. M., and R. G. Gibson. "The Treatment of Arthritis with a Lipid Extract of *Perna Canaliculus:* A Randomized Trial." *Complementary Therapies in Medicine* 6(1998):122–26.

Halpern, G. M. "Anti-inflammatory Effects of a Stabilized Lipid Extract of *Perna Canaliculus* (Lyprinol)." *Allergie & Immunologie* 32(2000)272–78.

———. "Recent Advances in Human Nutrition and the Science of Pleasure." Published in part in *EAACI Newsletter* 2–3(1999): 4–7.

Harris, W. S. "Omega-3 Fatty Acids and Serum Lipoproteins: Animal Studies." *American Journal of Clinical Nutrition* 65(1997): 1611S–1616S.

———. "Omega-3 Fatty Acids and Serum Lipoproteins: Human Studies." *American Journal of Clinical Nutrition* 65(1997):1645S–1654S.

Herold, P. M., and J. E. Kinsella. "Fish Oil Consumption and Decreased Risk of Cardiovascular Disease: A Comparison of

Findings from Animal and Human Feeding Trials." *American Journal of Clinical Nutrition* 43(1986):566–98.

Holgate, S. T., and M. K. Church. *Allergy.* London and New York: Gower Medical Publishing, 1993.

Hooper, S. "The Effect of Marine Oils on Markers of Thrombosis in the Blood of Healthy Females." Bachelor of Applied Science (Honours) Thesis, Department of Medical Laboratory Science (Haematology), Faculty of Biomedical and Health Sciences and Nursing, RMIT University, Australia, October 1998.

Hwang, D. H., P. S. Chanmugam, D. H. Ryan, M. D. Boudreau, M. M. Windhauser, R. T. Tulley, E. R. Brooks, and G. A. Bray. "Does Vegetable Oil Attenuate the Beneficial Effects of Fish Oil in Reducing Risk Factors for Cardiovascular Disease?" *American Journal of Clinical Nutrition* 66(1997):89–96.

James, M., R. A. Gibson, and L. G. Cleland. "Dietary Polyunsaturated Fatty Acids and Inflammatory Mediator Production." *American Journal of Clinical Nutrition* 71(2000)343S–348S.

Katan, M. B., P. L. Zock, and R. P. Mensink. "Effects of Fats and Fatty Acids on Blood Lipids in Humans: An Overview." *American Journal of Clinical Nutrition* 60(1994):1017S–1022S.

Kremer, J. M. "Omega-3 Fatty Acid Supplements in Rheumatoid Arthritis." *American Journal of Clinical Nutrition* 71(2000): 349S–351S.

Ludwig, D. S., K. E. Peterson, and S. L. Gortmaker. "Relation Between Consumption of Sugar-Sweetened Drinks and Childhood Obesity: A Prospective, Observational Analysis." *Lancet* 357(2001):505–08.

Mathews-Roth, M. M. "Carotenoids in Erythropoietic Protoporphyria and Other Photosensitivity Diseases." *Annals of the New York Academy of Sciences* 691(1993)127–38.

Natarajan, R., and J. Nadler. "Role of Lipoxygenase in Breast Cancer." *Frontiers in Bioscience* 3(1998)E81–88.

National Institutes of Health, Global Initiative for Asthma—Global Strategy for Asthma Management and Prevention NHLBI/WHO Workshop Report, March 1995, Publication No. 95-3659, January 1995.

Nestel, P. J. "Fish Oil and Cardiovascular Disease: Lipids and Arterial Function." *American Journal of Clinical Nutrition* 71(2000):228–31.

Rainsford, K. D., and M. W. Whitehouse. "Gastroprotective and Anti-inflammatory Properties of Green-Lipped Mussel (*Perna Canaliculus*) Preparation." *Arzneimittelforschung* 30(1980) 2128–32.

Shiels, I. A., and M. W. Whitehouse. "Lyprinol: Anti-inflammatory and Uterine Relaxant Activities in Rats, with Special Reference to a Model for Dysmenorrhea." *Allergie & Immunologie* 32(2000) 279–83.

Sinclair, A. J., K. J. Murphy, and D. Li. "Marine Lipids: Overview: New Insights, and Lipid Composition of Lyprinol." *Allergie & Immunologie* 32(2000):261–71.

Speed, A., and D. Zwar. "Introducing: The Ocean Mussel That Packs a Punch Against Arthritis Pain." *Bio/Tech News,* 1997.

Turcios, N. L. "What You Need to Know about Pediatric Asthma Pharmacology." *Contemporary Pediatrics* 18(2001):81–101.

Whitehouse, M. W. "Adjuvant-Induced Polyarthritis in Rats." In *CRC Handbook of Animal Models for the Rheumatic Diseases,* vol. 1, edited by R. A. Greenwald, and H. S. Diamond. Miami, Fla.: CRC, 1996.

———. "Non-NSAID Over-the-Counter Remedies for Arthritis: Which Are the Good, the Bad, the Indifferent?" SEADS/Inflammopharmacology Meeting, Georgia, May 1999.

Whitehouse, M. W., T. A. Macrides, N. Kalafatis, W. H. Betts, D. R. Haynes, and J. Broadbent. "Anti-inflammatory Activity of a Lipid

Fraction (Lyprinol) from the N.Z. Green-Lipped Mussel." *Inflammopharmacology* 5(1997):237–46.

Whitehouse, M. W., M. S. Roberts, and P. M. Brooks. "Over-the-Counter (OTC) Oral Remedies for Arthritis and Rheumatism: How Effective Are They?" *Inflammopharmacology* 7(1999):89–105.

# Glossary

***Acute*** Rapid in onset; severe, life-threatening. The opposite of persistent, chronic, or long-term.

***Arthritis*** Joint inflammation, a group of more than 100 rheumatic diseases that can cause pain, stiffness, and swelling in the joints. These diseases also affect other parts of the body, including structures such as muscles, bones, tendons, and ligaments, and some internal organs. The two most common forms of arthritis are osteoarthritis (OA) and rheumatoid arthritis (RA).

***Asthma*** A chronic inflammatory disorder of the airways in which many cells and cellular elements play a role—in particular, mast cells, eosinophils, T lymphocytes, neutrophils, and epithelial cells.

***Allergy*** An immediate or delayed immune reaction caused by an allergen—a substance such as dust, a drug, or other foreign material that causes an allergic reaction.

***Analgesic*** Agent that reduces pain without reducing consciousness.

**Antagonist** A drug that prevents or reverses the action of another drug.

**Anti-inflammatory** A substance that counteracts or suppresses inflammation. Swelling and redness are types of inflammation. There are two types of anti-inflammatory drugs: steroids, such as cortisone, and non-steroidal agents, such as aspirin.

**Antioxidant** A substance that neutralizes free radicals that break down the molecules and cells of the body.

**Arachidonic acid** An essential fatty acid that is a constituent of human cell membranes. It is also a precursor of inflammatory body chemicals.

**Autoimmune disease** A disease that arises from and is directed against an individual's own tissues.

**Cardiovascular system** The heart and blood vessels.

**Central nervous system** The main part of the nervous system; includes the brain and spinal cord.

**Chronic** Continuous or ongoing.

**Diabetes** A condition in which the pancreas produces too little or no insulin, the hormone that enables the cells to absorb glucose. The body becomes unable to use glucose, resulting in major diverse damages, mostly in blood vessels and sensory organs.

**Double blind** A type of drug trial in which people are divided into different groups. One group takes the experimental drug and other groups take different doses, the standard therapy, or placebo. Neither the researchers nor the people in the trial know who is taking what until the trial is over.

**Drug** According to the definition of the American Medical Association, "a chemical substance that alters the function of one or more body organs or changes the process of a disease." Drugs include prescribed medicines, over-the-counter remedies, and illicit drugs such as cocaine.

**Immunoglobulin E (IgE)** A class of antibody that is associated with allergy.

**Leukotrienes** Chemicals produced within the body that are responsible for initiating and extending the inflammatory process throughout the body. They develop through the lipoxygenase (LOX) pathway.

**Lipid** Any of a group of fatty substances including triglycerides (the main forms of fat in body fat), phospholipids (vital constituents of cell membranes), and sterols such as cholesterol.

**Placebo** A chemically inactive substance given instead of a drug. In clinical trials, placebos result in clinical improvement in up to 60 percent of patients.

**Prostaglandin** Any of a group of naturally occurring body chemicals, derived from fatty acids, that have a variety of effects, including contraction, inflammation, and damage to tissues.

**Symptom** A sign that the body is going through a process. A fever is a symptom of a more deep-rooted cause—namely, an infection. A rash is a symptom that the immune system is reacting to something such as allergens.

# Index

# INDEX

# INDEX

# INDEX

# ABOUT THE AUTHORS

*Georges Halpern, M.D., Ph.D,* is professor emeritus of medicine and of nutrition at the University of California, Davis, and Visiting Professor at the University of Hong Kong.

Dr. Halpern was born a French citizen in Warsaw, Poland, and attended medical school at the University of Paris. In 1964, he received his M.D. degree and was awarded a silver medal for his thesis. He subsequently qualified in nuclear medicine and was board certified in internal medicine and allergy. In 1992, he received his Ph.D. degree, with highest honors and jury honors, from the Faculty of Pharmacy at the University of Paris XI.

He was recently promoted to the rank of Commander in the French National Order of the Mérite Agricole for his original contributions to French cuisine and enology.

Dr. Halpern has published twelve books, many book chapters, original papers, and hundreds of reviews and abstracts. He has lectured in seventy-four countries. In 1985, he was awarded the Medal of Vermeil by the city of Paris for his outstanding contributions to medicine, dedication to patients, and personal achievements.

Dr. Halpern is a Fellow of the American Academy of Allergy, Asthma, and Immunology, and of twenty-six other academies and scientific societies. He resides in Portola Valley, California.

*Krista Edmonds, Ph.D,* who collaborated on the book, received her degree in the psychology of women from Columbia Pacific University in 1989. She has been actively involved in alternative medicine and the exploration of human potential for over thirty years. In addition, she led a project on the Lunar Surface Geologic Experiment during the Apollo Program. She founded and has successfully run her own company in organizational development consulting and training for twenty years. She has written five books, including *Dancing in the Face of the Wind: Healing Women's Fears of Success,* to be published in 2001. She lives in New Mexico.